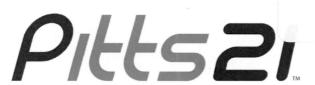

"OUR METHOD"

Time and Space in
Passive Self Ligation
Treatments

Prologue: **Dr. Thomas Pitts**

Dr. Federico Nappa Severino
Dr. Alfredo Nappa Aldabalde
Dra. Marisa Villalba Hidalgo

ESPARTA FORMACIÓN ODONTOLÓGICA
www.espartaformación.com

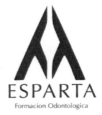

ESPARTA
Formacion Odontologica

ISBN: 978-9915-40-298-7
Edition: YDEAS S.R.L.
Cover: Designed by Federico Nappa
ALL RIGHTS RESERVED © 2020

ISBN: 978-9915-40-298-7

Forward / Prologue

As a practicing orthodontist for over 50 years, an orthodontic teacher/professor, and a colleague of the authors for many years, I can unequivocally recommend this book to all orthodontists and hope they embrace its message.

I have always believed that patients deserved beautiful smiles, in addition to straight teeth. Creating good occlusions and straightening teeth has become easy for most orthodontists, but getting consistent great smile and facial esthetics simultaneously, on most orthodontic cases, has eluded many of my colleagues. Dogma is pervasive in our profession. As a result, many orthodontic finished smiles, "miss the mark". This book will show you how to more easily "hit the mark".

I have been working on "Pitts Esthetic Discipline" in orthodontics for many decades. Criticism has been frequent as the profession ponders some of the innovations, I had a hand in. Diagnosing and treating to esthetically optimal results, requires a different skill set and processes than those needed to make good occlusions, and "straighten teeth". Diagnosing from the "outside/in" to esthetic standards has been novel in orthodontics. The Latin American authors, of this book, picked up on this and have now given us a playbook, that they developed of their renditions, of our protocols. Thanks to orthodontists like these authors, we now have orthodontic "artists", stepping up and researching these concepts.

The authors also show some disruptive innovations to speed up treatment, including Pitts21, Pitts Broad wires, ultra-soft NiTi's in 18x18 and 20x20. The "engage early" square wire AW approach incorporates biologically friendly forces. They show how this square wire appliance with light forces, is making orthodontics a much more enjoyable experience for the patients.

The authors, unlike the majority of orthodontists who write about biomechanics, and show little consideration to enhancing smile and facial esthetics, show how and why enhancing the esthetics is so important to the patient.

The Nappa family has been at the forefront of our specialty, in subscribing to "disruptive innovations" that make sense. They have helped to confirm that we can make extraordinary esthetics and very efficient treatment with newer philosophies and biomechanics, and still have great occlusal function.

The authors have taken precious time to write the first book on these progressive esthetic and efficient orthodontic techniques with light forces. They have become great teachers of these techniques and valued contributors to our journey. My hat's off to Drs. Nappa, and Dra. Marisa Villalba Hidalgo for their commitment to "Progressive Orthodontic Treatment".

I am very proud that they would ask me to do a forward for this exciting new book. Please read this material with an open mind. Don't let the dogma sneak in.

Thomas Pitts DDS, MSD

Clinical Professor University of Nevada Las Vegas, Orthodontic Program
Private practice of orthodontics, Reno, Nevada

Dedication

Infinite thanks:

To our families, the support of our lives.

To our dear teachers, for so many lessons they left us.

To the educational institutions that sponsor our courses.

To O.C. Orthodontics Distributors and Vendors.

To Dr. Tom Pitts and his teaching teams.

To our partners in programming.

To our office assistants.

To the dear teaching groups where we participate.

To the patients who have trusted our professional work.

To the great driving forces behind all of this, the reason for the classes…, this book is yours,

colleagues, so that you either enjoy it … or endure it …

Dr. Federico Nappa Severino
Dr. Alfredo Nappa Aldabalde
Dra. Marisa Villalba Hidalgo

Dedication of the authors to the Book of the Pandemic

You have been a special book in a special moment of our lives and of humanity itself. We love you as a child conceived and born under those particular circumstances.

Now, son, you must walk across the world with your successes and mistakes; then it will be the time of your life, your way ...

Good luck, dear son. Book of the Pandemic.

Topic index

Prologue by Thomas Pitts DDS, MSD 3
Dedication. 5

Section 1... 8

Time and space in aesthetics
Chapter 1 ... **Introduction** 9
Chapter 2 ... **Patient 1** 22
Chapter 3 ... **Patient 2** 57

Section 2... 70

Stages in Simultaneous Biomechanics
Chapter 4 ... **Introduction** 71
Chapter 5 ... **Patient 3** 86
Chapter 6 ... **Patient 4** 94
Chapter 7 ... **The Role and Origin of the Dysfunction in Treatments** 103

Section 3... 157

Asymmetries and Asymmetric Biomechanics
Chapter 8 ... **Introduction** 172
Chapter 9 ... **Patient 5** 168
Chapter 10 ... **Patient 6** 186

Section 4... 200

Time and Space of the 3rd. Molars
Chapter 11... **Introduction** 201
Chapter 12 ... **Patient 7** 219
Chapter 13 ... **Patient 8** 239

Chapters 4, 7, and 8, have sequences of 3 treatments using Pitts21.
Chapters 7 and 11 have sequences of 2 treatments using H4.

SECTION 1

TIME AND SPACE IN AESTHETICS

Section 1
Time and space in aesthetics
Chapter 1
Introduction

Innovation distinguishes between a leader and a follower"
Steve Jobs 1955-2011
Outstanding American computer scientist and entrepreneur, founder of Apple.

Time and its inevitable passing, confronted us again, but this time in a different way, with the challenge of the blank page that, at the same time, captivates us and earns our respect.

Now the challenge is to develop a book that shows different *Pitts21* topics and cases with some common threads such as time, space and our method.

Because of very characteristics of the publication and the new times we live in, we have cut out the words, and increased the images of the cases.

We will not include definitions of time or space here, two "frenemies" that appear in our lives, sometimes tiptoeing into more or less inconsequential anecdotes, while, on occasion, they are the cornerstone of philosophical and religious conception of our life.

In these times it is common for both, colleagues and patients, to be very active in technological networks, with their great advantages in the immediacy and plurality of data collection.

As in life itself, there is a counterpart and consequence of hyperconnectivity and hyper information that is not the same as knowledge, and a true mental chaos can be caused. *(Figs. 1 to Fig. 4)*

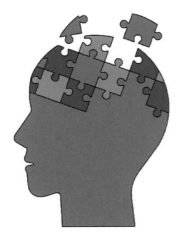

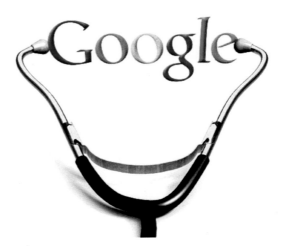

1

2

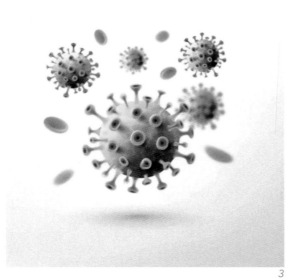

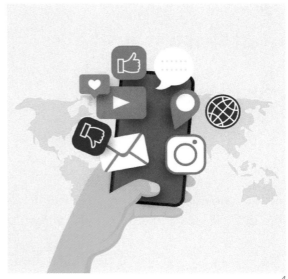

3

4

Perhaps one of the main challenges for an educator in an online classroom course or when writing a book, is getting one's mind in order and convey a methodology; in no way this means that we own the truth, or that there are no other ways of teaching and learning. *(Fig. 5)*

We believe in the ENDLESS LEARNING GEN ...

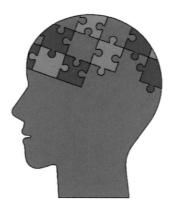

5

Method. Way to reach a goal.

The method means that organization of the subject matter that makes it more effective in its use.
John Dewey (1859-1952)
American pedagogue, psychologist and philosopher.

Let's imagine that a treatment is a trip, it can be shorter or longer and present more or less obstacles in order to reach the destination. On that trip we will use one or more vehicles that will carry us from the beginning to our final destination.

The starting point, place, date and time in our treatments is the diagnosis **D**, and the objectives are the arrival.

To move from one to another there will be a certain plan **P**; one or more vehicles **V** with someone

who drives and must know their operation, mechanics and route to be covered (biomechanics) **B**.
(Fig. 6, 7, and 8)

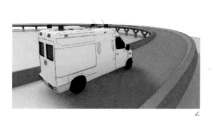

6

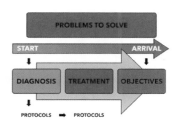

7

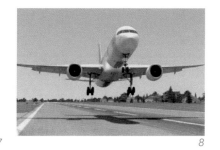

8

Therefore, the method is to know the diagnosis **D**, establish a treatment plan **P** and the therapeutic vehicles **V** to carry it out, and finally, put that plan into practice with certain management or biomechanics **B**.

Although there are several diagnostic areas, generally, the requirements of our patients relate to two of them, the aesthetics and also the time or duration of the treatments. *(Figs. 9 to 14)*

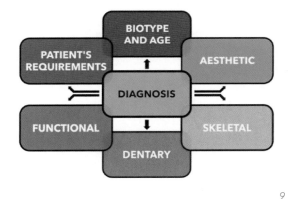

9

"NO WIND IS FAVORABLE
FOR THOSE WHO DO NOT KNOW
WHERE THEY ARE GOING"

SENECA

10

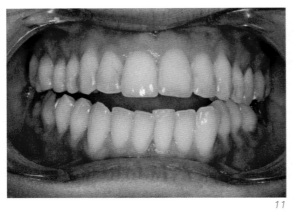
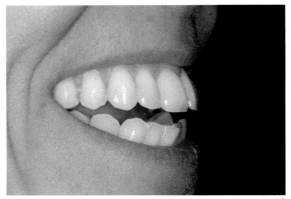

11

12

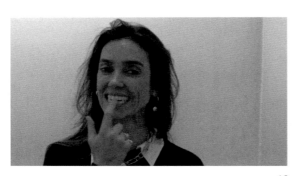
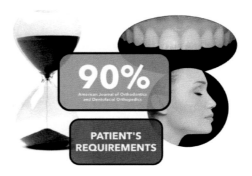

13

14

In this book, we will present successful cases using *Pitts21* passive self-ligating. But both, the vehicles themselves and the different stages of the method, have disruptive components.

A disruptive technology or activity changes a pre-existing product dramatically. *(Fig. 15 and 16)*

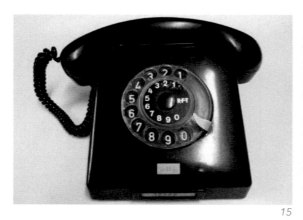
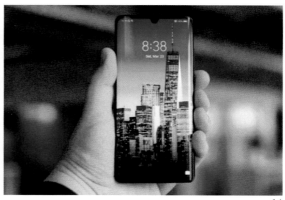

15

16

To be disruptive, you must first think differently and, if possible, in a simple way so that, in this activity, orthodontics is understood both, by patients and professionals in the specialty. *(Fig. 17 and 18)*

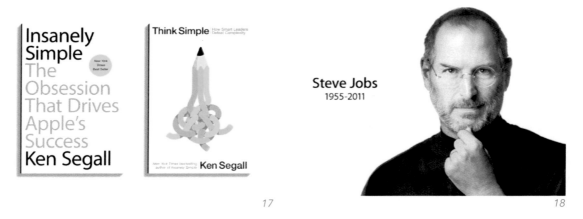

"Innovation distinguishes between a leader and a follower". Steve Jobs (1955-2011)

Within the diagnosis and treatment objectives, the aesthetics plays a fundamental role in satisfying the demands of our patients. *(Fig. 19 to 22)*

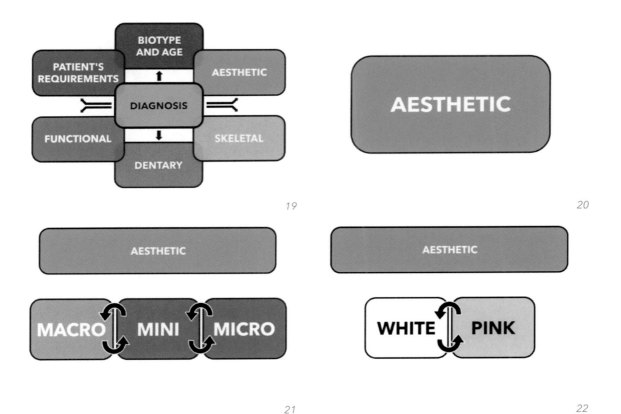

All of these areas can be improved with treatments:

- Orthopedics
- Functional orthopedics
- Orthodontics
- Surgical orthodontics
- Periodontics
- Dental operative restorations
- Facial aesthetic procedures

Here we will expose facial and oral images, including some videos, of 4 patients in their pre- and post-treatment; these cases will be appreciated in different sections of this book.

Patient A – *(Figs. 23 to 49)*

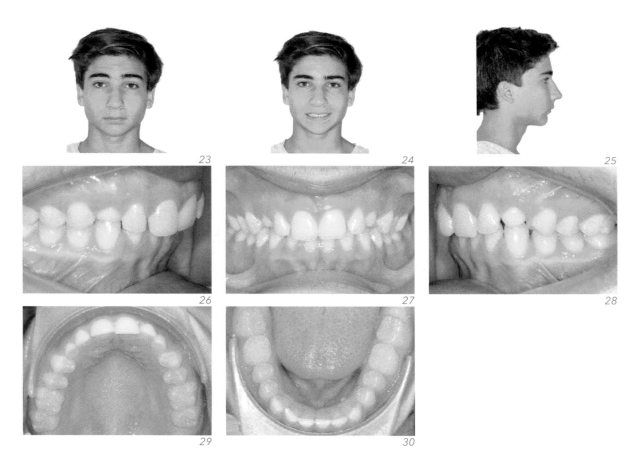

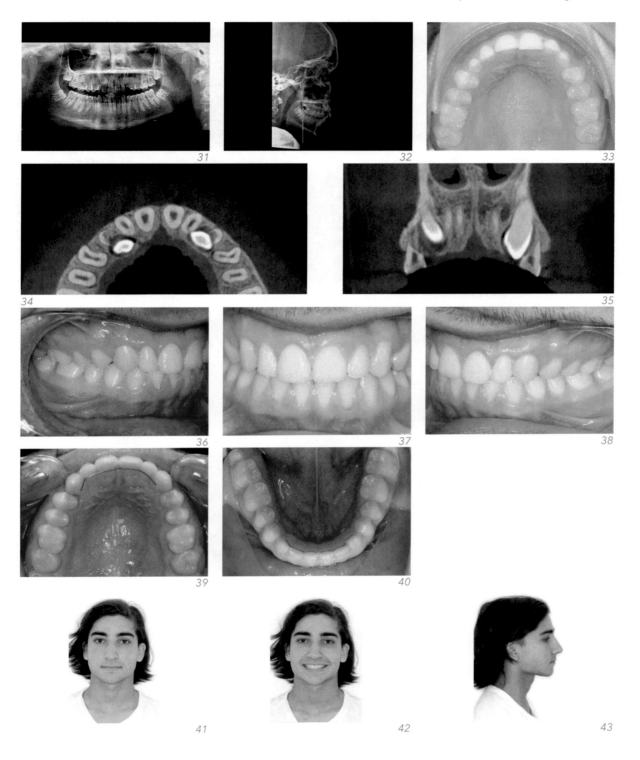

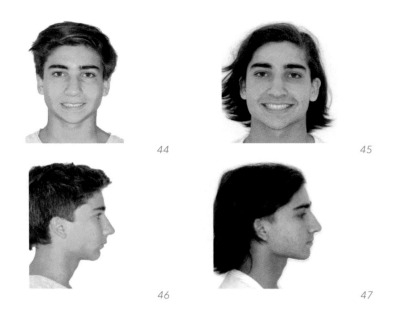

44

45

46

47

Patient B - *(Figs 48 to 68)*

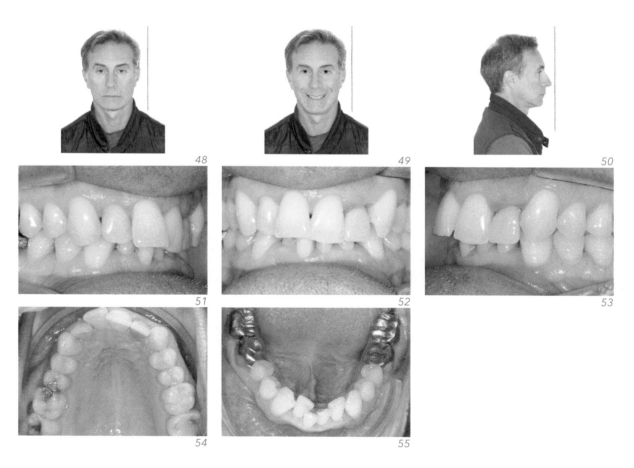

48

49

50

51

52

53

54

55

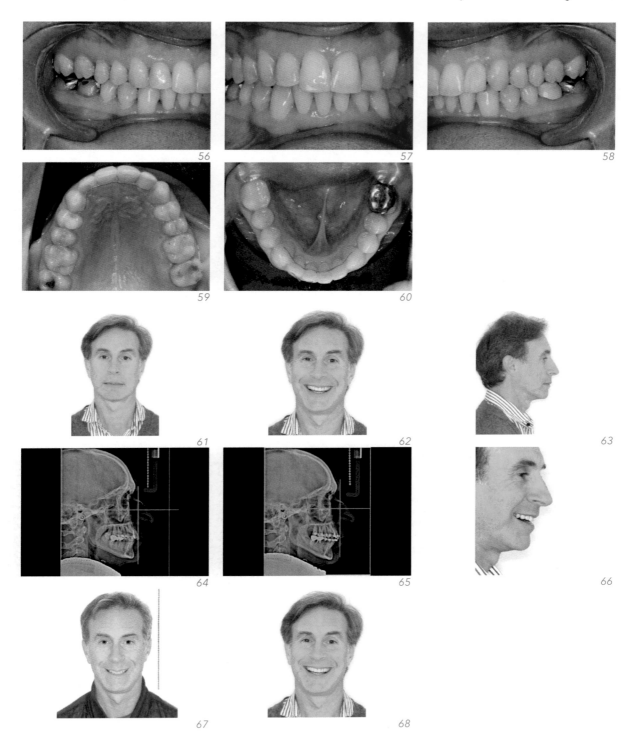

Patient C - *(Figs. 69 to 83)*

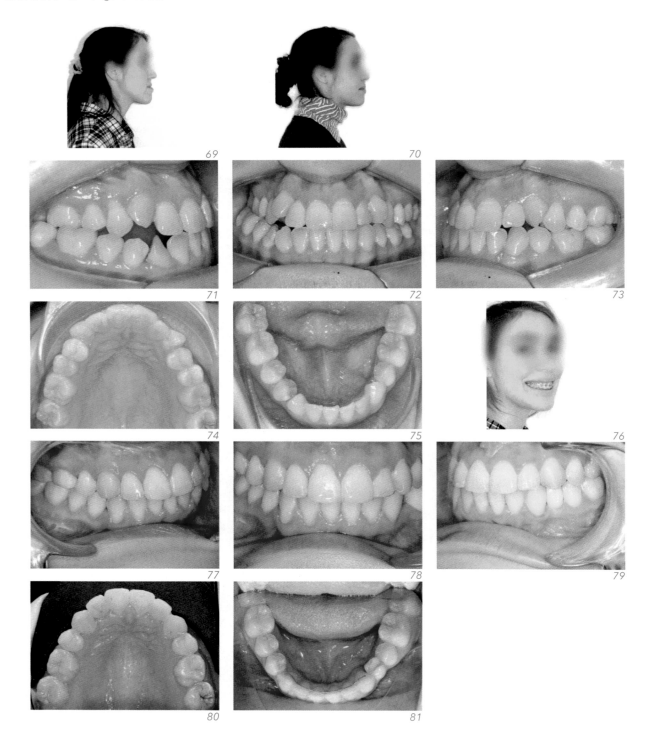

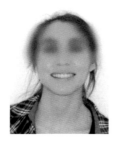

82

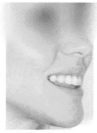

83

Patient D - *(Figs. 84 to 107)*

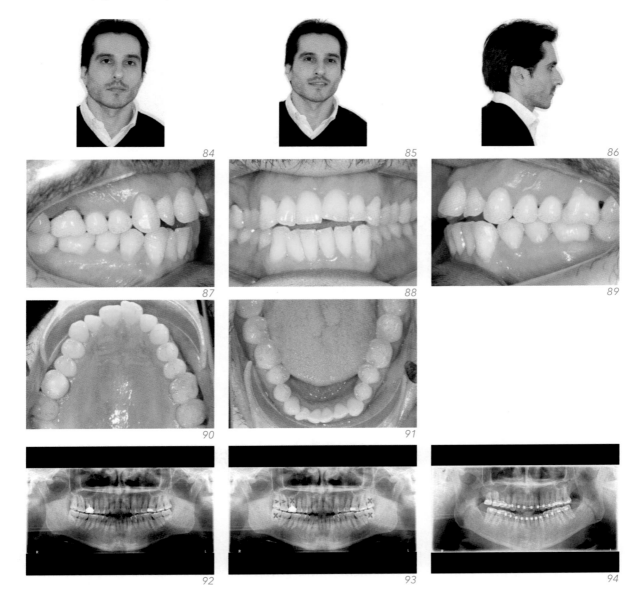

84

85

86

87

88

89

90

91

92

93

94

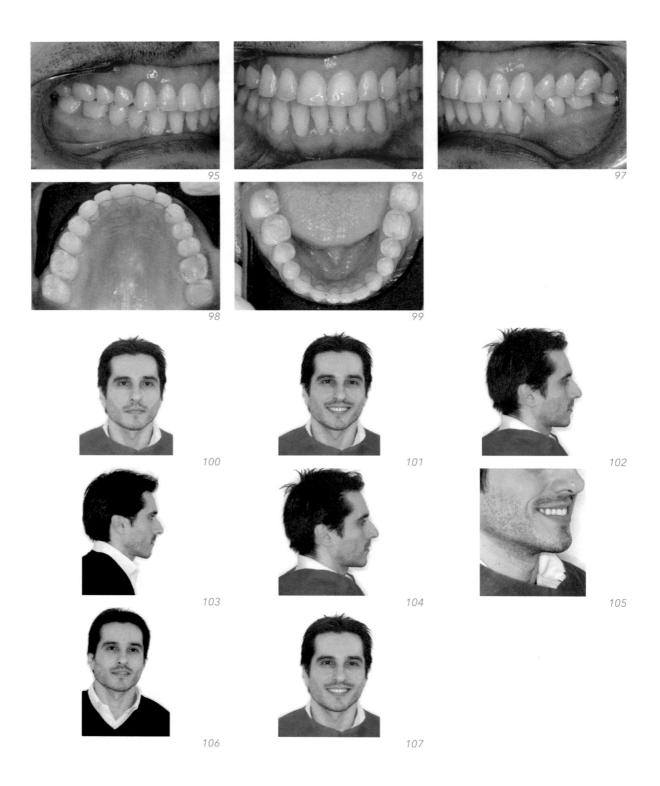

In these next chapters, when presenting cases, we will address various aesthetic aspects based on the concepts of **Dr. Thomas Pitts,** but applied with our method. *(Figs. 113 to 115)*

SMILE DESIGN AND AESTHETIC EVALUATION

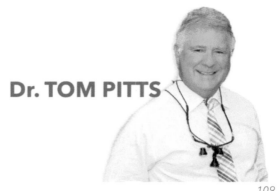

Dr. TOM PITTS

108

109

1) **FULL DENTAL MASS**

2) **FULL LIP / CHIN SOFT TISSUE**

3) **INCISOR INCLINATION**

4) **V.I.P. / VERTICAL INCISOR DISPLAY**

5) **S.A.P. / SMILE ARC PROTECTION**

6) **BROAD ARCH - 12 TOOTH SMILE**

7) **CHEEK CURVATURE**

8) **UPPER MIDLINE vs LIP PHILTRUM**

9) **OCCLUSAL PLANE SYMMETRY**

10) **PRESENCE OF PAPILLA**

110

Section 1
Aesthetics time and space
Chapter 2
Patient 1

Anyone who keeps the ability to see beauty never grows old
Frank Kafka 1883-1924
Prague, Czech Republic

9 out of 10 patients, that is, 90%, go to our daily practice for AESTHETIC REASONS, and this highlights the GREAT IMPORTANCE of aesthetics in treatments and the main concern of solving malpositioned teeth.

Within this category (malpositioned teeth), the "problem" itself appears with variants, but with a common background: the discrepancy between tooth and bone (sectorized or more generalized insufficient space in one or both arches).

Orthodontically, this is called "negative dental discrepancy" and can be the cause of different clinical "manifestations".

Main clinical manifestations
produced by the negative dental discrepancy

NEGATIVE DENTAL DISCREPANCY

DENTAL MALPOSITIONS VARIANTS, MAINLY - CROWDING

TEETH RETENTIONS

DENTAL AND FUNCTIONAL ASYMMETRIES

Taking into account these "manifestations", how many times have you asked yourself the following question:

"Is extraction the only way to deal with negative discrepancy?"

When dealing with the lack of space issue for good teeth positioning in teens and adult treatments, not in all cases but in many, the first question that arises is: **to extract or not to extract?**

TO EXTRACT **TO NOT EXTRACT**

To answer this question, we will look at a case, where the treatment was performed through the implementation of "**our DPVB method**" (a clinical protocol based on a **D** Diagnosis, a Planning according to the said diagnosis, and the use of a specific **P.V** therapeutic vehicle to finally reach to the **B** Biomechanical protocols).

This **DPVB** clinical protocol will present a logical order, which will help you to systematize any treatment that comes your way.

The constant implementation of this protocol in our daily practice can become a habit and thus, it is possible to approach any treatment, be it of greater or lesser complexity, with great simplicity.

With this systematic approach, you will be able to reach the final destination of the treatment with clinical efficacy and efficiency, with and easy and timely resolution.

DPVB METHOD
D   **DIAGNOSIS**
P.V   **PLANNING / THERAPEUTIC VEHICLE**
B   **BIOMECHANICS**

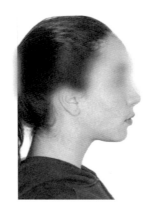
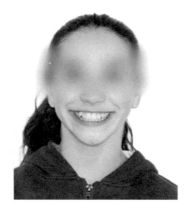
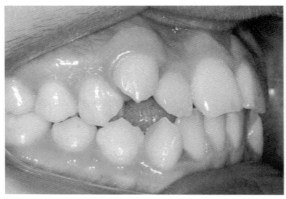
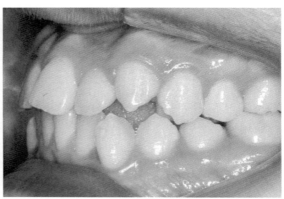
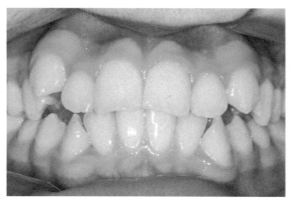
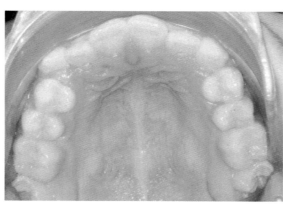
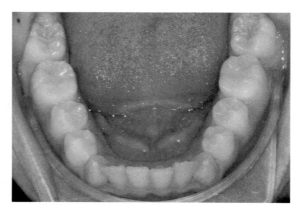

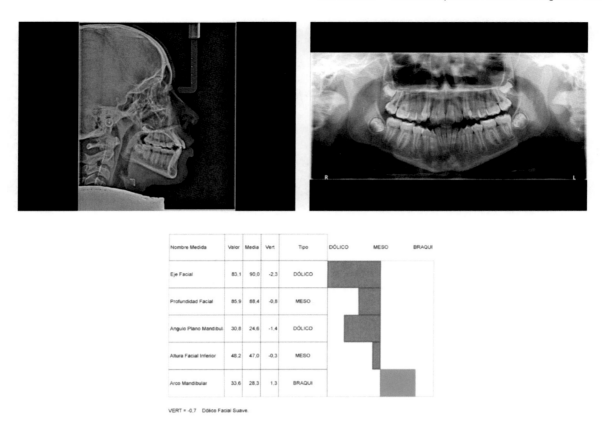

Nombre Medida	Valor	Media	Vert	Tipo	DÓLICO	MESO	BRAQUI
Eje Facial	83,1	90,0	-2,3	DÓLICO			
Profundidad Facial	85,9	88,4	-0,8	MESO			
Angulo Plano Mandibul.	30,8	24,6	-1,4	DÓLICO			
Altura Facial Inferior	48,2	47,0	-0,3	MESO			
Arco Mandibular	33,6	28,3	1,3	BRAQUI			

VERT = -0,7   Dólico Facial Suave.

After showing the extra and intraoral photographs, the lateral and panoramic radiographs, along with the biotype analysis, we will begin to implement and describe of our **DPVB** method, step by step. Let's start with the DIAGNOSIS:

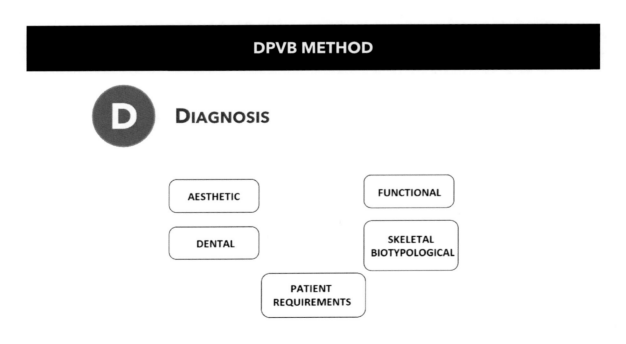

From the diagnostic point of view, we are going to consider 6 factors:

- **AESTHETIC**
- **DENTAL**
- **FUNCTIONAL**
- **SKELETAL / BIOTYPOLOGICAL**
- **PATIENT REQUIREMENTS**

Aesthetic analysis and patient requirements

Regarding these diagnostic factors, as we mentioned at the beginning of this chapter, 9 out of 10 patients will have aesthetics as their main requirement. Dr. Sarver classifies the aesthetic analysis, and divides it into 3:

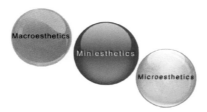

- **MACROESTHETICS**
- **MINIESTHETICS**
- **MICROESTHETICS**

For practical purposes, and to continue simplifying the daily work at the clinic, we recommend that you make this diagnosis in a visual way as Dr. Dwight Frey does by assigning colors (diagnostic visualization) and NOT by using numbers or cephalometric values that can be hard to remember later.

Dr. Dwight Frey performs this assessment using 3 colors to which we add the yellow color, considering the time as a determining factor for certain modifications.

VISUALIZACIÓN DIAGNOSTICA BASADA EN 4 COLORES

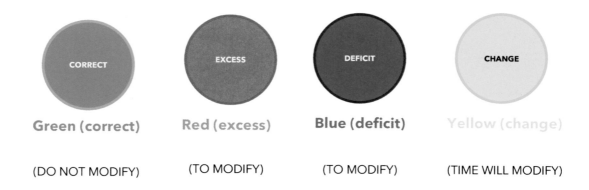

Green (correct)	Red (excess)	Blue (deficit)	Yellow (change)
(DO NOT MODIFY)	(TO MODIFY)	(TO MODIFY)	(TIME WILL MODIFY)

MACROESTHETICS

- VERTICAL PROPORTIONS

- HORIZONTAL PROPORTIONS

- LIP CLOSURE

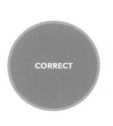
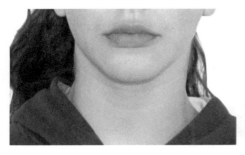
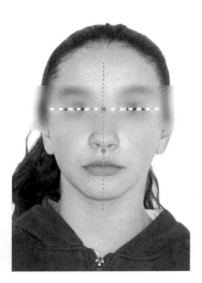

- NASOLABIAL ANGLE

- NASAL PROJECTION (NASAL TIP)

- PROFILE

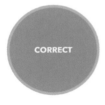
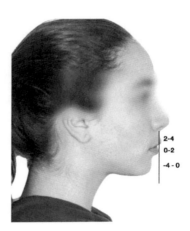

In **MACROAESTHETICS,** in the frontal view, we have to take into account:

- VERTICAL PROPORTIONS

- HORIZONTAL PROPORTIONS

- LIP CLOSURE

And, on the *lateral or profile view*, we have to take into account:

- Nasolabial angle.

- Mentolabial angle.

- Nasal projection (Nasal *Tip*).

- Upper lip, lower lip, and chin projection. Ideal aesthetic proportions in the adult and the projected sub-nasal vertical line.

Taking into account all this for clinical simplification and its eventual diagnostic visualization, we will assign the **GREEN** color which means "**DO NOT MODIFY**" because it is correct.

When we analyze the lateral X-ray, and making an aesthetic diagnosis based only on the position of the upper incisor with respect to **GALL** (**G**oal **A**nterior **L**imit **L**ine) line of Andrews, we observe that the upper incisor is proclined (ideally the buccal surface of the upper incisors should be vertical and parallel to this reference line). As this is an inclination excess, so we will assign the red color, which means **"TO MODIFY".**

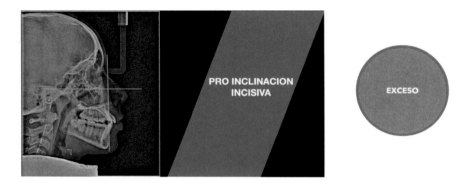

Quoting Dr. David Sarver again, *"It is important to correct what is altered, but more important is to maintain what is correct"*, so we will have to resolve that proclination without altering, for example, the nasolabial angle, which is correct (**GREEN**).

MINIESTHETICS

- VISUALIZATION OF INCISORS

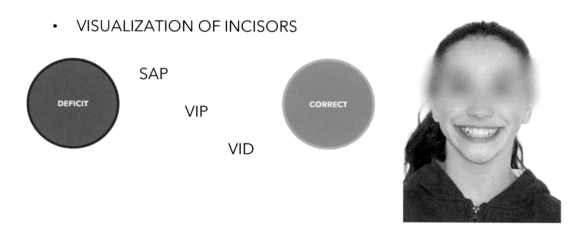

- BUCCAL CORRIDORS

- GINGIVAL DISPLAY

- SMILE HEIGHT

In **MINIAESTHETICS**, we have to take into account:

- VISUALIZATION OF INCISORS AND RELATED TO SAP, VIP AND VID.

- FACIAL MIDLINE.

- BUCCAL CORRIDORS.

- GINGIVAL DISPLAY.

- SMILE HEIGHT.

The word "**aesthetics**" derives from the Greek voices and means "Sensation", "Perception", which is why, at this point, the patient requirements take more than a leading role for the decision making, as there may be differences in perceptions.

We can see that there are aspects related to mini-aesthetics that are correct, so we assign them the **GREEN** color (DO NOT MODIFY); those that are in deficit (the smile) are assigned the **BLUE** color (TO MODIFY).

"The ideal vertical display of upper incisors, both at rest and during smiling, constitutes one of the most important assessment aspects in facial mini-aesthetics".

Visualization of incisors in **GREEN**, taking into account the "today" status of the patient as there are changes that are age-related, as seen in the chart (Fig. 1).

AVERAGE DENTAL DISPLAY AT REST (MM)[7]		
	Maxillary Central Incisor	Mandibular Central Incisor
Less than 30	3.4	0.5
30 - 40	1.6	0.8
40 - 50	1.0	2.0
50 - 60	0.5	2.5
More than 60	0.0	3.0

Taking into account the "tomorrow" status of the patient, the SAP (**S**mile **A**rc **P**rotection), VIP (**V**ertical **I**ncisor **P**osition) and VID (**V**ertical **I**ncisor **D**isplay) play a fundamental role in the **P**lanning/Therapeutic **V**ehicle.

The **buccal corridors** are correct, despite presenting a pronounced dentoalveolar imbalance in both arches (which can narrow the upper arch creating the so-called "black corridors" of the smile).

The **gingival display** in "today" status of the patient is correct, but here you will have to consider the information of Fig. 1 related to the cruel passage of time, which is, the "tomorrow" where the soft tissues increase the flaccidity, and the result is that they show less of the maxillary and more of the mandibular teeth.

SMILE HEIGHT

Low	less than 75 % of display of the tooth crown.
Medium	between 75 % and 100 % of display of the tooth crown.
High	100 % of display of the tooth crown, and up to 3 mm of gingival display.
Gingival	When the gingival display is more than 3 mm. (It can be due to different factors).

"These smile heights can be altered by various factors, including the cruel passage of time."

MICROESTÉTICA

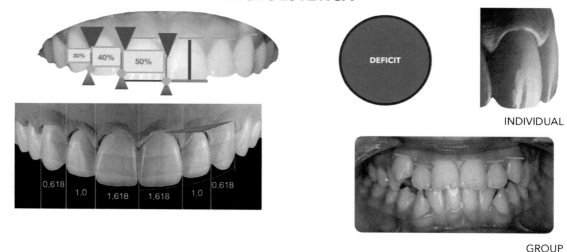

INDIVIDUAL

GROUP

- RELATED FACTORS
- DENTAL ANALYSIS

When we analyze **MICRO-AESTHETICS**; we have to consider that it is a dental assessment and analysis, both individually and by group.

- At this point, all factors related to MAINTAINING or MODIFYING proportions of white aesthetic (tooth) and pink aesthetic (gingiva) will be important.

- Here we clearly see a **DEFICIT** in that aspect.

Up to here, the patient underwent an AESTHETIC Diagnosis:

- MACRO-AESTHETICS

- MINI-AESTHETICS

- MICRO-AESTHETICS

SKELETAL / BIOTYPOLOGICAL ANALYSIS

By Rickets, the lateral X- ray and its cephalometry, evidences that this case is a mild dolichocephaly biotype with a lower incisor proclination.

The Andrews line called **GALL** (**G**oal **A**nterior **L**imit **L**ine) is a reference line on which we rely for our dental proclination diagnosis. Base on this reference line and the lateral X- ray analysis, we observe that the upper incisor is proclined.

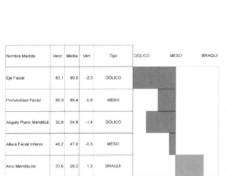

Nombre Medida	Valor	Media	Vert	Tipo	DÓLICO	MESO	BRAQUI
Eje Facial	83,1	90,0	-2,3	DOLICO			
Profundidad Facial	86,9	86,4	-0,8	MESO			
Angulo Plano Mandibul.	30,8	24,6	-1,4	DÓLICO			
Altura Facial Inferior	46,2	47,0	-0,3	MESO			
Arco Mandibular	33,6	26,3	1,3	BRAQUI			

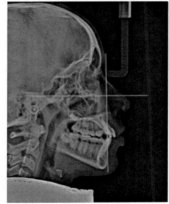

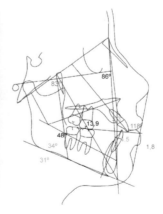

This analysis becomes a factor to be considered for the planning and subsequent execution of certain biomechanics, which may be conditioned by a specific skeletal / biotypological situation.

UPPER BASAL

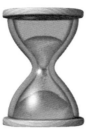

UPPER DENTOALVEOLAR

_____

LOWER DENTOALVEOLAR

LOWER BASAL

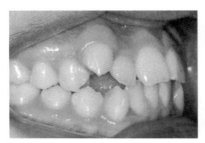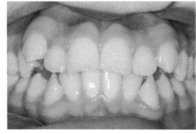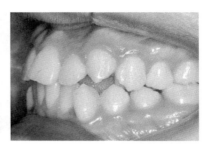

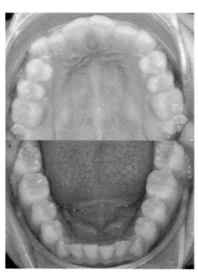

Occlusal analysis

The frontal view of this case with poor anterior guidance shows a dentoalveolar narrowing caused by a functional imbalance, both of the upper arch and lower arch, forming what we call the HOURGLASS in the dentoalveolar area.

The lateral view shows the Class I molar and canine relationships.

The upper and lower occlusal views show the existing negative discrepancy, and as we mentioned in the beginning of this chapter, one of the clinical "manifestations" produced by negative dental discrepancy are the dental malpositions in their different variants.

Given that 90% of the SUCCESS of a treatment is based on a correct **D**iagnosis, it is time to apply the Diagnosis to the second point of our "DPVB" method, which is the **P**lanning / Therapeutic **V**ehicle.

PLANNING / THERAPEUTIC VEHICLE

In planning, we will analyze certain points that have arisen from the **D**iagnosis, such as: **dolycho biotype + incisor proclination + negative dental discrepancy + poor anterior guidance**, and we must add to them ALL the factors that we **DO NOT HAVE TO MODIFY (GREEN).**

The factors listed in previous paragraphs led us to ask ourselves: are we before a premolar extraction case?

Since the patient had a high AESTHETIC requirement, the extractions were not compatible with some of the 14 keys that Dr. Tom Pitts considers for aesthetics.

Top 14 keys of Dr. Pitts for aesthetics

1. FULL DENTAL MASS.

2. PROPER INCLINATION OF INCISORS / CUSPIDS.

3. SMILE ARC CURVATURE.

4. INCISAL AND GINGIVAL DISPLAY.

5. 12-TOOTH SMILE.

6. AESTHETIC AND FUNCTIONAL ARCH SHAPE.

7. MICROESTHETICS.

8. MINIAESTHETICS.

9. FULL UPPER LIP.

10. NICE SOFT CHIN PROJECTION.

11. INCISAL PLANE SYMMETRY.

12. UPPER MIDLINE.

13. RESTORATIVE CONSIDERATION FOR POOR MORPHOLOGY.

14. SOFT FACIAL TISSUE ENHANCEMENT.

Therapeutic Vehicles

- Pitts21 passive self-ligating.

- Archwires.

- Intermaxillary elastics.

"For the effective and efficient achievement of the objectives that we set, it is necessary to put this therapeutic vehicle triad to work together".

Pitts21 passive self-ligating

As orthodontists, we have always used rectangular slots (.022" x .028" and in some cases with a larger measure) in our treatments. First with round cross-section archwires for alignment and leveling, and later with rectangular cross-section archwires (x.025") for the expression of Tip, Torque and Rotation.

This slot / archwire gauge relationship caused an extension of our clinical times because the transmission of these movements shows up late in the treatment.

At one point, life crossed our paths with Dr. Thomas Pitts again, but this time was with the H4 bracket, which, while it continued to have a rectangular slot, it also presented a UNIQUE variant at that time which we believed was essential for the daily practice (less clinical time); The depth of the bracket slot was reduced, going from .022" x.028" slot from edgewise to a .022" x .026" slot. Keeping in mind that the rectangular archwires continued to be x.025", the dimensional relationship between bracket slot and arch gauge changed substantially. Additionally, there was more control over the movements (something highly questioned in passive self-ligating).

This first reduction allowed us to have a clinical improvement due to the Archwire/Slot relationship.

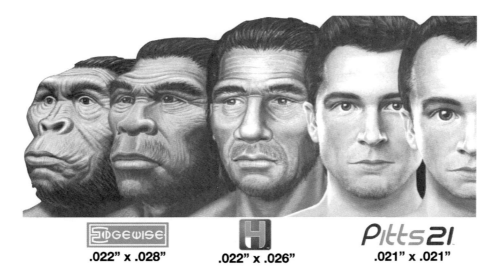

Then, Dr. Pitts went a step further and created the Pitts21 Bracket in 2 varieties (metallic and the more current, Clear21), whose slot has the distinctive feature of being square in the anterior sector from 3 to 3 (.021" x .021"), maintaining a rectangular slot for posterior sectors (.021" x .023" Premolars - .021" x .024" Molars). This detail provides exceptional control of the anterior teeth while giving greater freedom of movement to the posterior teeth.

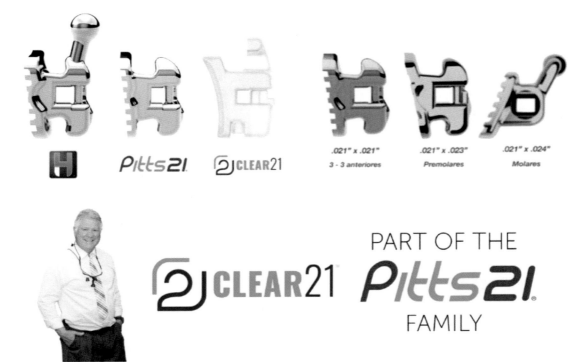

In Pitts21 bracket, the classic dimensions of a rectangular slot and rectangular cross-section archwires for the expression of the Tip-Torque and Rotation change to a square slot and square cross-section archwires for the same movements.

This relationship provides a 3D control and the earliest expression of Tip, Torque, and Rotation (early engagement), with 30-40% less force.

4 contact points for the transmission of torque with .020" x .020" archwire in 0.21" x .021" slot, with only 4° archwire/slot relationship of free play.

TIP

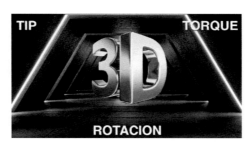

TORQUE

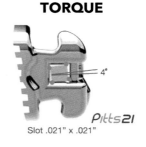

ROTATION

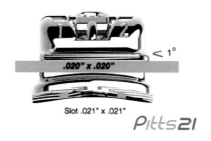

Prescriptions

The three-dimensional control, and so, the palatobuccal inclination of the teeth, is very important in treatments, because it plays a main role when we want to achieve certain aesthetic and functional objectives.

To introduce ourselves to the selection of the prescription, I believe it's convenient to refer to the second and third keys mentioned by Dr. Andrews in his study of models belonging to patients with ideal occlusions and that have not been treated orthodontically.

- The second key refers to the mesiodistal angulation that was observed in the models. In a bracket, the expression of this **angulation** is called "TIP".

- The third occlusion key described by Dr. Andrews refers to the inclination palato or lingual buccal of dental crowns. In a bracket, the expression of this **inclination** is called "TORQUE".

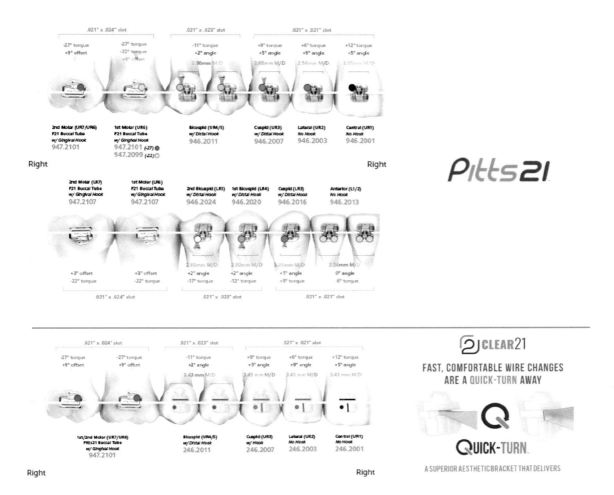

Selection of upper incisor bracket prescription

To select the upper incisors bracket prescription, it is convenient to remember that in Pitts21 we have only one prescription, which we can transform into two simply by turning the bracket in 180 degrees.

To select the prescriptions, it must be remembered that our diagnosis will be mainly from the aesthetic point of view, taking as reference the pre-treatment upper incisor and its relationship to the GALL, and taking into account the mechanics (elastics, extractions, etc.) that influence such positioning.

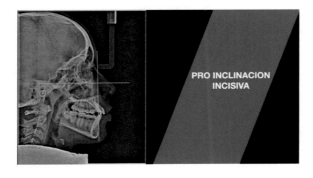

With all this in mind, there will be cases in which we will need a different torque in the upper arch: where we will opt for a variant in the placement, that is, we will give the bracket a 180 degree turn to obtain negative torque (this turn can be individually or by group).

180-degree turn - upper 2-2 = **Flipped**

180-degree turn - upper 3-3 = **Flocked**

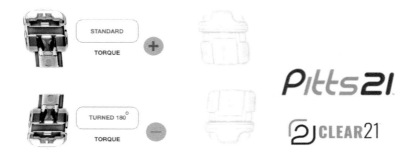

There will also be cases in which we will need a positive torque in the anterior inferior sector, which has a 2-2 negative torque (keep in mind that the canines have a positive torque). As in the upper arch, we can opt for a 180-degree turn (this turn can be individually or by group).

Archwires

In this point, we are going to analyze the archwire variants that will be used in the Pitts philosophy.

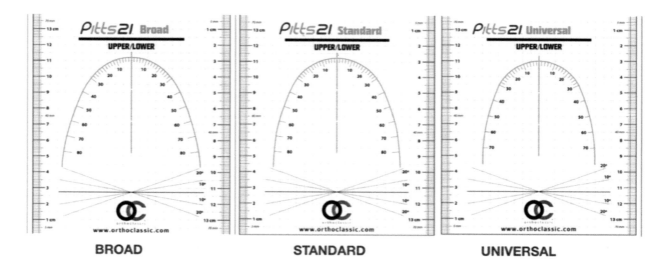

Remember that the archwire diagram in orthodontics is composed, among other factors, by the intercanine distance and the intermolar distance, and when analyzing the archwire diagram of the H4/Pitts21-Clear21 system, we observe these varieties:

A. BROAD

B. STANDARD

C. UNIVERSAL

These 3 variants have a similar intercanine distance and differ only in intermolar distance; the Pitts Broad has the largest.

- Here there is no upper or lower archwire; it is used interchangeably.

- Regardless the diagram, this is the archwire option menu that will be used in Pitts21 or Clear21.

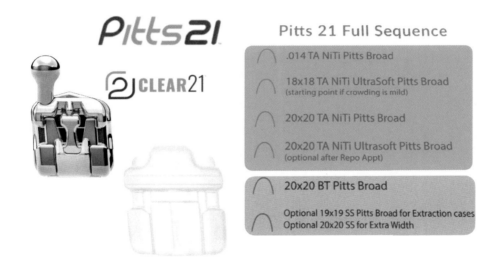

We are going to divide this option menu into two large groups according to the material:.

NON FORMABLES archwires		They correspond to the NiTi TA archwires (**T**hermo **A**ctivated **N**ickel **T**itanium)
FORMABLES archwires		They correspond to the BT archwires (Beta Titanium) and SS arches (Steel).

TIEMPOS EXPRESADO EN SEMANAS   Slot .022" x .028"

0	10	20	30	40	50	60	70

FASE	INICIAL		TRABAJO		DETALLES Y FINALIZACION
SECCION	.014	.018	.014 x .025	.018 x .025	.019 x .025
MATERIAL	NiTi	NiTi	NiTi	NiTi	Acero
CONTROL DE TORQUE	No Control	No Control	28.77°	13.78°	10.88°
CONTROL DE ROTACION	8.47°	6.09°	1.85°	1.85°	1.85°
CONTROL DE TIP	4.29°	2.15°	4.29°	2.15°	1.62°

TIEMPOS EXPRESADO EN SEMANAS   *Pitts21*   Slot .021" x .021"

0	6	12	18	36

FASE	INICIAL	TRABAJO		DETALLES Y FINALIZACION
SECCION	.014	.018 x .018	.020 x .020	.020 x .020
MATERIAL	NiTi	NiTi	NiTi	Beta Titanio, TMA o Acero
CONTROL DE TORQUE	No Control	14.20°	4.18°	4.18°
CONTROL DE ROTACION	4.44°	1.92°	0.64°	0.64°
CONTROL DE TIP	3.83°	1.92°	0.55°	0.55°

In this table, we clearly see the favorable arch / slot relationship for the early expression of tip, torque and rotation movements when using Pitts21 compared to brackets with rectangular slots.

As can be seen in the Pitts21 table, all movements are achieved using NiTi archwires with light forces.

Intermaxillary elastics

We will have to take into account that for a correct and rapid resolution of the case, the use immediate intermaxillary elastics (ILSE) is necessary.

We can classify them into two groups:

- BY DIAMETER

- BY FORCE

In biomechanical protocols and in the remaining clinical cases, this point will be addressed in more detail in order to understand the combinations of diameter, force and their placement.

DIÁMETER

FORCE

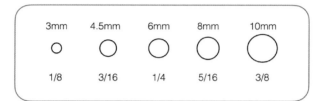

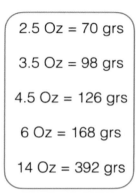

1 inch = 25, 4 mm

1 Oz = 28 grs

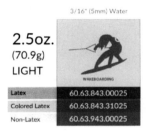

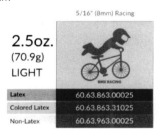

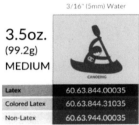

Bonding planning

After the diagnosis, planning the bonding is a fundamental part for the success of the treatment.

Developing the ability of selecting the bracket prescription and bonding of tubes and brackets will be key to achieving a beautiful smile (WOW), and a good functional occlusion, pointing out that both objectives are not in conflict with each other.

Extraordinary Esthetic Goals Do Not Have to Conflict with Occlusal Goals *(Dr. Tom Pitts)*

SAP (Smile Arc Protection)

From a frontal view, in an ideal smile arc, when smiling, the incisal edges of upper teeth (incisors and canines) are parallel to the curvature of the lower lip.

The first definition of the smile arc was limited to the upper incisor and canine sector and, also, it was exclusively valued from the frontal view; but the view of the arc of the complete smile also includes posterior teeth and is complemented by their vision, at 45 degrees.

To create this ideal arch (WOW smile), the upper brackets are positioned more gingivally than in traditional techniques and, also, divergent in relation to the cusps and incisal edges of the teeth in the upper jaw.

Thus, the orthodontic archwire is not parallel to the occlusal plane (Straight Arch reference) but mesially divergent with respect to said plane, in which it generates a certain edging in a clockwise direction.

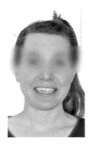 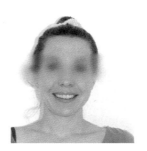

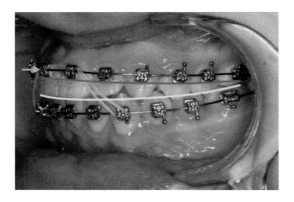 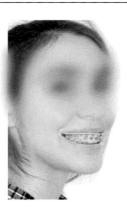

Another important aspect of MINI-AESTHETICS is the pre and, especially, post-treatment torque of upper incisors; in their final position, factors such as its pre-treatment inclination, selection of prescription, bonding on the buccal surface of the incisors, and biomechanics may influence to the initial pro or retroclination, influence. Incisor torque can be assessed clinically and also on a profile X-ray.

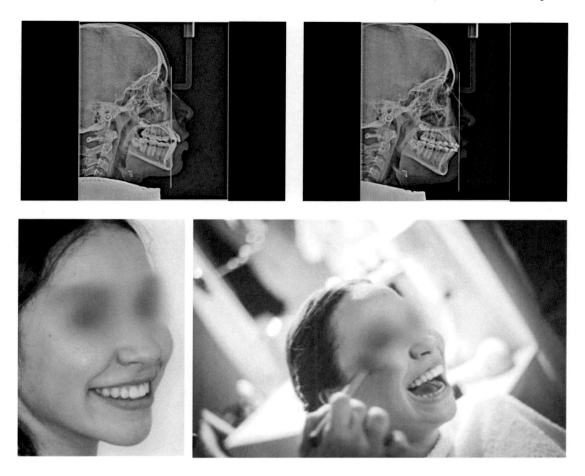

ACRONYMS		
SAP	SMILE ARC PROTECTION	ARCO DE LA SONRISA
VID	VERTICAL INCISOR DISPLAY	EXPOSICIÓN VERTICAL INCISIVA
VIP	VERTICAL INCISAL POSITION	POSICIONAMIENTO VERTICAL INCISAL (SUPERIOR)
	The latter considers the **VID** and the upper incisor inclination.	

Last but not least, we have to make all this "machinery" work in a very particular way, NOT in a sequential way, but through an "early activation" with **_simultaneous biomechanics_**. This way, most of the corrections will be achieved with the early stages of the NiTi archwires, and the steel archwires will be left exclusively for extraction cases and proper space management.

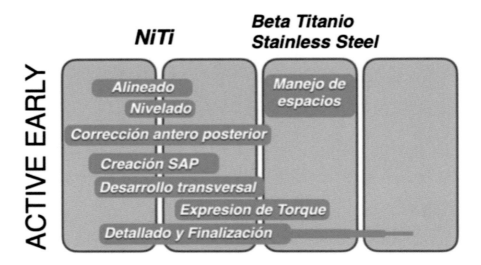

In this last point of our method, we will simply apply the corresponding biomechanical protocols to reach the objectives set for our patient:

Remember that the aesthetic is a main requirement for our patient.

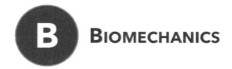 **B** **BIOMECHANICS**

BIOMECHANIC PROTOCOLS

The challenge we faced with this patient was that technically, it was a case for 4 premolar extractions.

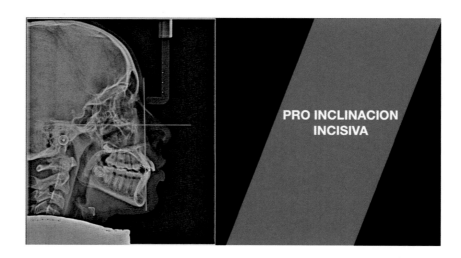

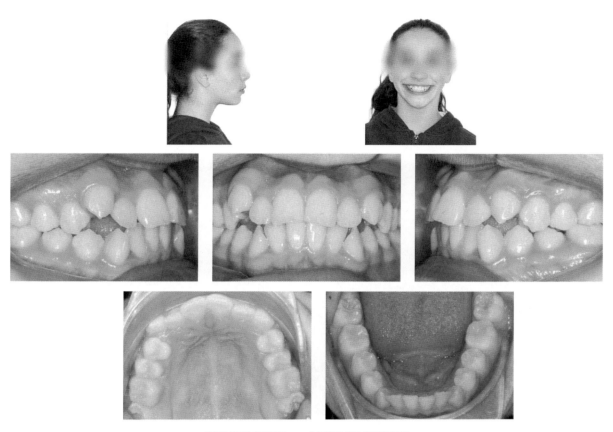

REMEMBER ... LESS IS MORE

LESS EXTRACTIONS

SIMPLE MECHANICS

BUT, HOW TO ACHIEVE INCISOR RETRACTION WITHOUT PREMOLAR EXTRACTIONS?

INCISOR RETRACTION

WITHOUT PREMOLAR EXTRACTION

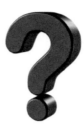

SIMPLY... BY FOLLOWING THESE BIOMECHANICAL PROTOCOLS

1) **BROAD ARCHWIRES**

2) **FLIPPED / FLOCKED BRACKETS**

3) **GINGIVAL BONDING**

4) **TORQUE CHAIN**

---

1) BROAD ARCHWIRES

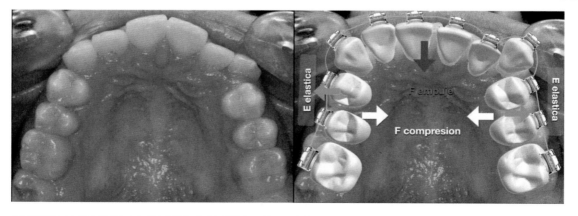

THE TRANSVERSAL DEVELOPMENT IS ALSO KEY TO ACHIEVE THE CORRECTION OF THE ANTERIOR SECTOR.

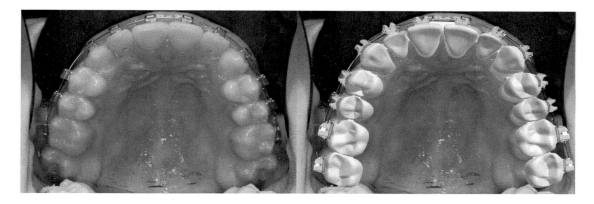

BROAD ARCHWIRE .018 x .018" NiTi Ultra Soft

2)   FLIPPED / FLOCKED BRACKETS

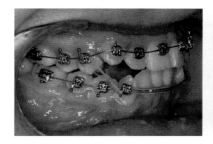 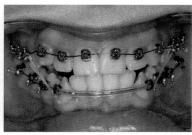 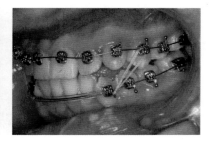

Remember that the bracket prescription arises from the aesthetic diagnosis, the pre-treatment position of the upper incisor, as well as the mechanics that influence said positioning.

We need a negative torque in the anterior superior sector of the patient.

This is due to its incisive proclination added to the anterior discrepancy that will be partly resolved by the transversal development and parlay by proclination. We bonded Flipped brackets, with a 2-2 180-degree turn. We placed the Flocked only in those cases with very inclined canines.

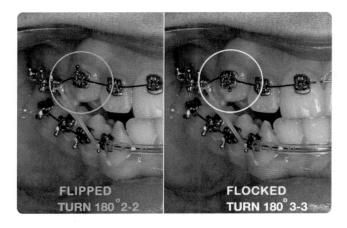

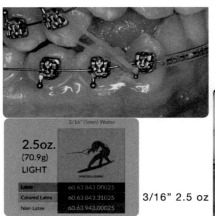

Elásticos cortos
inmediatos (ILSE)

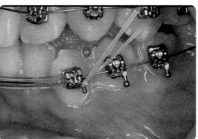

3/16" 2.5 oz

BIOMECHANICAL ADVICE: In cases that have a negative anterior discrepancy with incisive proclination and the lower canines in front of the incisors, place a bypass in the incisor sector and **ILSE** (**I**mmediate **L**ight **S**hort **E**lastics) of 3/16" diameter and 2.5 oz of force with a Class III vector to verticalize the lower canines; then bond the into incisors.

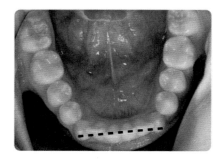

3)   GINGIVAL BONDING

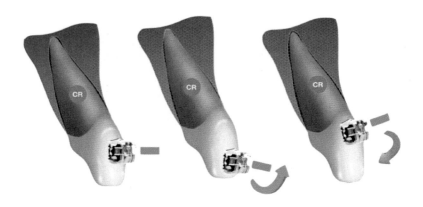

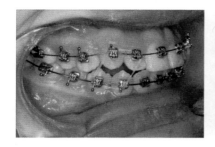 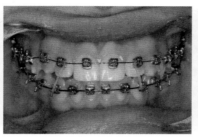 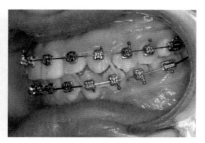

Due to the anatomy of the buccal surface of the incisors, the more gingival bonding results in the bracket slot to be arranged "as if looking up", and thus contributes to the expression of the negative torque of the rotated bracket.

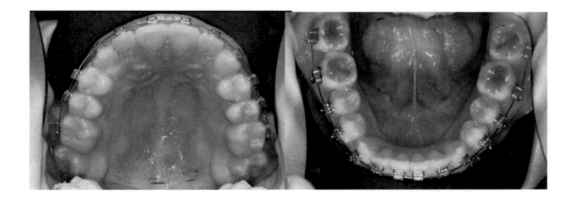

Since this is a dolycho patient with little anterior guidance, the disarticulations (a very important part of achieving the treatment goals) are placed in posterior sectors.

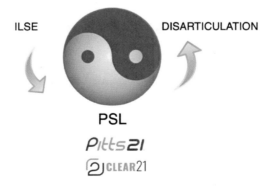

KEY COMPONENTS TO ACHIEVE MAXIMUM EFFECTIVENESS IN TREATMENTS. AN INDISSOLUBLE TRIAD

- IMMEDIATE SHORT ELASTICS (ILSE)

- DISARTICULATIONS (Anterior or Posterior)

- PASSIVE SELF-LIGATING Bracket Pitts21 / Clear21

BIOMECHANICAL ADVICE: squeezing exercises will also be part of a functional therapy because it exercises the closing muscles. It is done as follows:

60 squeezes (feel a contraction of the masseter and temporalis muscle) as quickly as possible, six times a day.

Ejercicios Squeezing

TERAPIA MIOFUNCIONAL
  - Masetero

  - Temporal

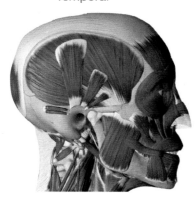

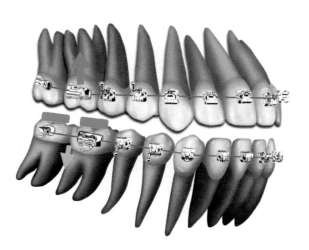

Among others, these are some of the objectives of the disarticulation:

- Enhance the action of the archwires for intra-arch movements.

- Enhance the action of the elastics for inter-arch movements.

- Vertical selective control in:

  - Open bite (small posterior intrusion)

  - Overbite (extrusion of posterior sectors)

OBJECTIVES	• ENHANCE THE ACTION OF THE ARCHES (INTRA ARCADE)
	• TO ENHANCE THE ACTION OF THE ELASTICS (INTRA ARCADE)
	• VERTICAL SELECTIVE CONTROL (OPEN BITE - COVERED BITE)

4) TORQUE CHAIN

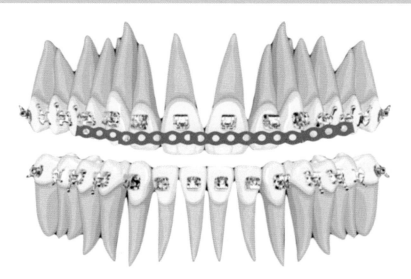

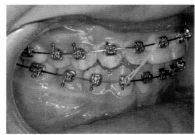 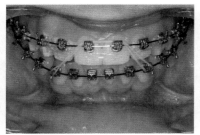 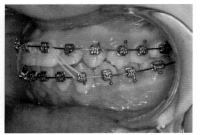

With Pitts21, we only use it in the .018 x .018" from teeth # 14 to 24
8 links of continuous chain

... and this is how we simply achieve the aesthetic objectives with function, in just 9 months.

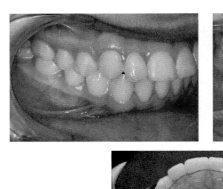
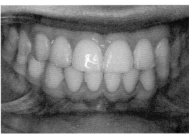
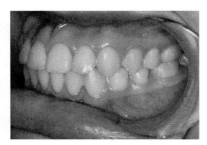

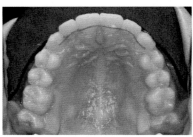
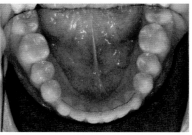

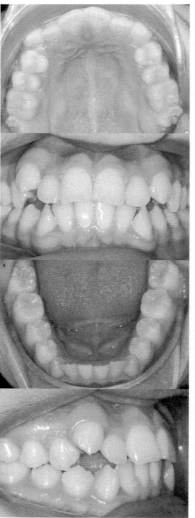
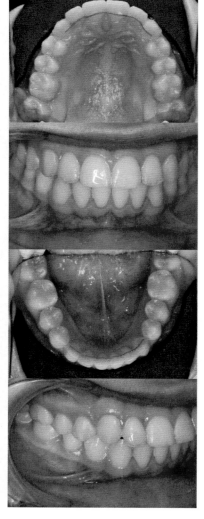

The aesthetic philosophy of Dr. Pitts aims to **create** a completely natural anatomical smile.

As mentioned in planning, the 14 aesthetic factors (top 14 smile Aesthetics) must be taken as a reference.

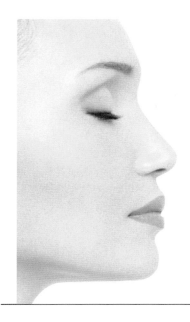

TOP 14 SMILE AESTHETICS

1 FULL DENTAL MASS

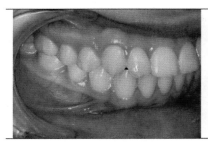 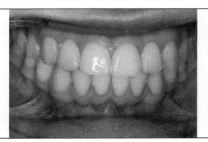 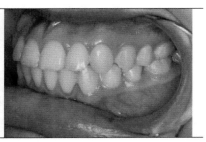

2 PROPPER INCISOR INCLINATION

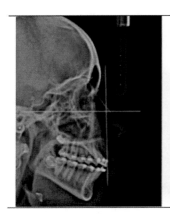 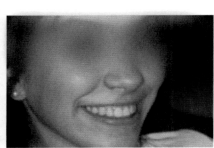 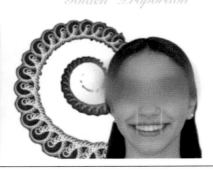

3 / 4 / 5 12 TOOTH SMILE / GINGIVAL DISPLAY

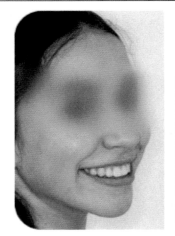

"Smile Arc"

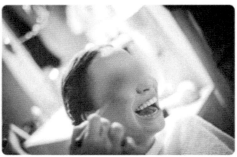

6 BROAD ARCH FORM IN Pm and M

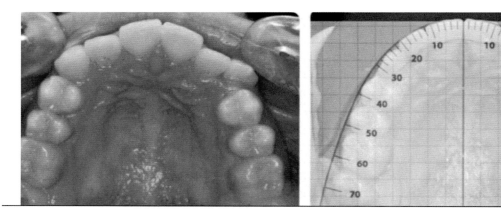

| PRE TREATMENT | FINAL |

7 MICROESTHETICS

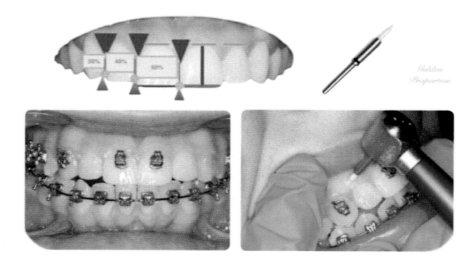

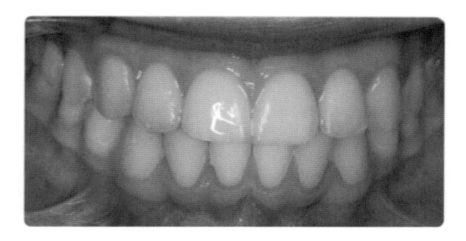

"Rounded and softened Incisal edges"

8 MINIESTHETICS

9 / 10 CHIN PROJECTION FULL LIPS

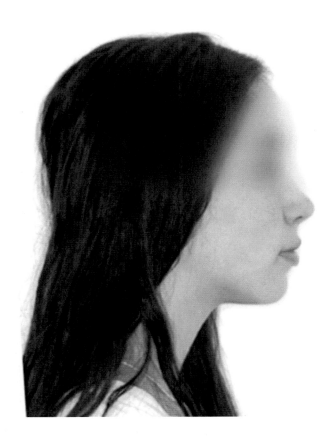

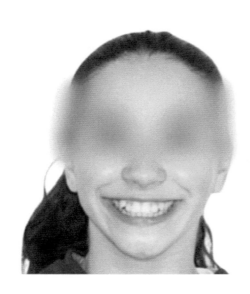 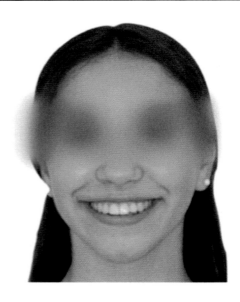

13 / 14

RESTORATIONS WERE NOT NECESSARY. IT HAD GOOD MORPHOLOGY. AND THE IMPROVEMENT OF THE FACIAL AESTHETICS IS IN SIGHT.

Extraordinary Esthetic Goals Do Not Have to Conflict with Occlusal Goals *(Dr. Tom Pitts)*

Section 1
Aesthetic time and space
Chapter 3
Patient 2

"One who smiles rather than anger is always stronger" **Zen quote**

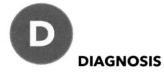

DIAGNOSIS

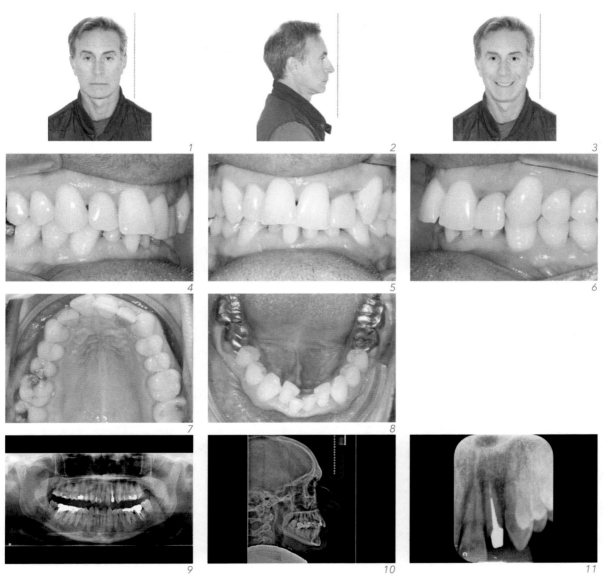

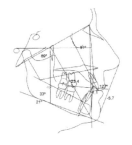

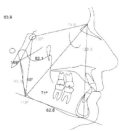

12   13

This case was an adult patient whose main requirements were:

- Treatment that will not exceed 12 months
- Dental aesthetics improvement
- Avoid the extraction of premolars (an option that had been suggested at another clinic)

As mentioned above, we have applied the diagnostic classification by **Dr. Dwight Frey** in almost 100% of cases:

- **Green** (correct)
- **Red (excess)**
- **Blue (deficit)**
- Yellow (change) *

* The current assessment will change (improving or worsening) over time (growth, changes in soft tissues, etc.)
The color system provides a quicker vision of the present status of our patient to which we add the (yellow) color to represent the change that can improve or worsen the initial status due to growth or the simple and inevitable passage of time.

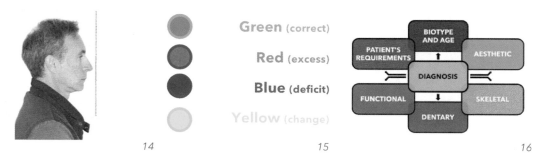

14   15   16

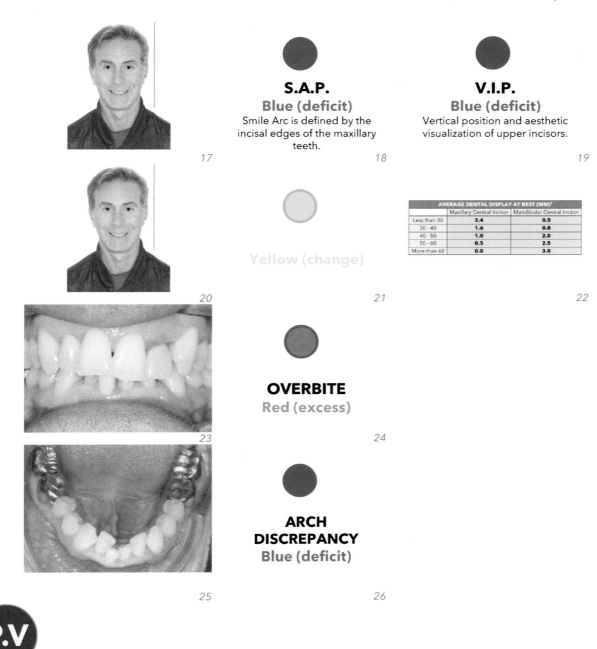

S.A.P.
Blue (deficit)
Smile Arc is defined by the incisal edges of the maxillary teeth.

17

V.I.P.
Blue (deficit)
Vertical position and aesthetic visualization of upper incisors.

18

19

Yellow (change)

AVERAGE DENTAL DISPLAY AT REST (MM)²		
	Maxillary Central Incisor	Mandibular Central Incisor
Less than 30	3.4	0.5
30 - 40	1.6	0.8
40 - 50	1.0	2.0
50 - 60	0.5	2.5
More than 60	0.0	3.0

20

21

22

OVERBITE
Red (excess)

23

24

ARCH DISCREPANCY
Blue (deficit)

25

26

P.V

PLANNING / THERAPEUTIC VEHICLE

The correction of the overbite includes an antero-superior extrusion to improve vertical exposure of upper incisors (VIP) which is clearly insufficient and will worsen with the passing of time. *(Figs. 17 to 24)* This approach constitutes a disruption in the traditional plans to correct occlusal problems.

As seen in figures 27 and 28, there are different alternatives for the correction of the overbite and, clearly, we opted to flatten the curve of Spee, which requires the bonding of tubes and brackets, similar to those seen in figure 29.

SOLUTION PATHWAY	
1.	"FLATTENING" OF THE CURVE OF SPEE
2.	ANTEROSUPERIOR INTRUSION / GINGIVAL SMILE?
3.	MANDIBULAR ADVANCEMENT
4.	INCISOR PROINCLINATION
5.	REHABILITATION OF POSTERIOR SECTORS OF THE MOUTH

27

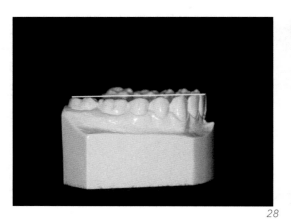

28

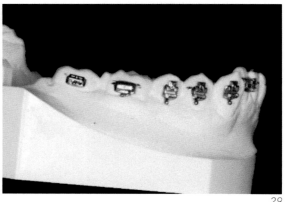

29

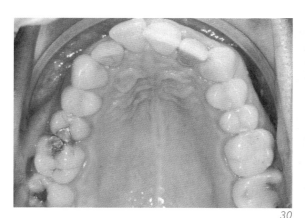

30

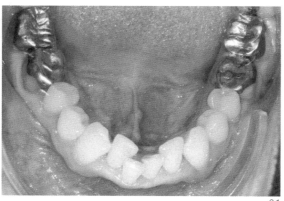

31

The negative discrepancy observed in both arches *(Fig. 30 and 31)* would be solved with a development of arch (Broad Pitts), in diameter and perimeter, along with some interproximal reductions (IPR). The goals of the treatment were:

- Protect macro aesthetics

- Maintain upper incisor inclination **(green)** *Figs. 32 to 34*

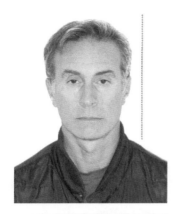

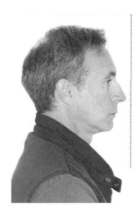

32

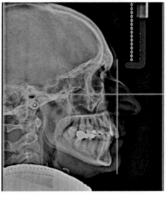

33

34

V THERAPEUTIC VEHICLE/S

The Pitts21 PSL brackets and tubes were used with "Flipped" superior prescription where incisor brackets are rotated 180° (negative torque to protect the correct pre-treatment inclination of his upper incisors (correct) and due to the marked negative dental discrepancy).
Said therapeutic vehicle was used in anterior disarticulation, elastics (ILSE) and archwire progression detailed in the biomechanics of the case.

B BIOMECHANICS

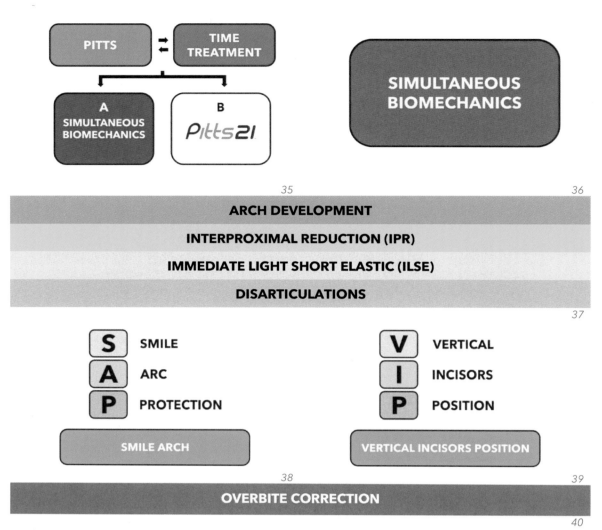

SIMULTANEOUS
BIOMECHANICS

PITTS ⇌ **TIME TREATMENT**

A SIMULTANEOUS BIOMECHANICS

B Pitts21

35

36

ARCH DEVELOPMENT

INTERPROXIMAL REDUCTION (IPR)

IMMEDIATE LIGHT SHORT ELASTIC (ILSE)

DISARTICULATIONS

37

S SMILE

A ARC

P PROTECTION

SMILE ARCH

V VERTICAL

I INCISORS

P POSITION

VERTICAL INCISORS POSITION

38

39

OVERBITE CORRECTION

40

In view of the magnitude of the negative dental discrepancy (- 9mm in the lower arch) and the periodontal status of the patient, the arch development began, seeking a very low load-deflection.

LOAD DEFLECTION RATE FACTORS
1) ARCHWIRE ALLOY
2) ARCHWIRE CROSS-SECTION
3) ARCHWIRE LENGTH
4) INTERBRACKET DISTANCE
5) FRICTION
6) INCIDENCE ANGLE (THE CAR AND THE ROAD)

41

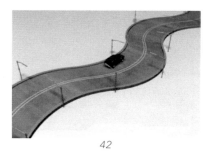

42

The biomechanical factors that influence this relationship are shown in *Figs. 41 to 42*.

In our lectures when we make the "car and road" reference, we want to express that by ignoring the inclusion of a tooth or using simple lock washers (Baby Eyelets), we are reducing the incidence angle in curves (malpositions) just like the Formula 1 drivers do.

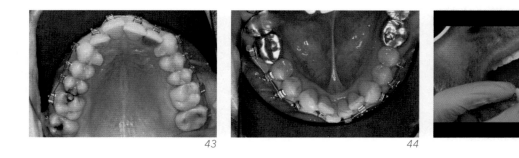

43   44   45

This purpose is set forth in *Figs 43 to 45* with .014" **Niti Broad Pitts** archwires.

Also, note the palatal disarticulations of teeth # 13 and 23 with the 3/16" 2.5 oz Class III immediate light short elastics (ILSE) aiming for a slight verticalization of teeth # 33 and 43. *Figs. 46 to 48*

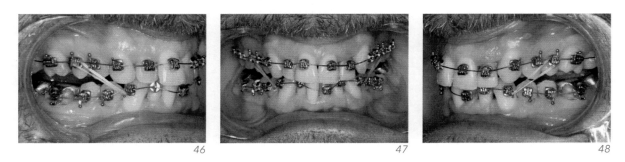

46   47   48

Five weeks later, using the same archwire, tooth 41 is connected, and a lock washer (Baby Eyelet) is bonded to it. *(Figs. 49 to 51)*

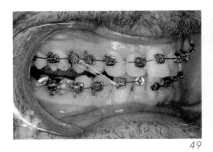
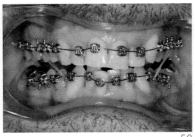
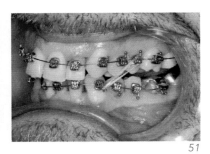

49   50   51

As the arch development began to improve, it was time (4 months of treatment) to include the upper and lower second molars with .018 x .018" **NiTi Ultra Soft Pitts Broad** archwires.

The use of said archwire has innumerable advantages in combination with a .021 x .021" bracket slot in the anterior sector, from canine to canine, and we usually use it for a variety of situations shown in *Figs. 52 to 62.*

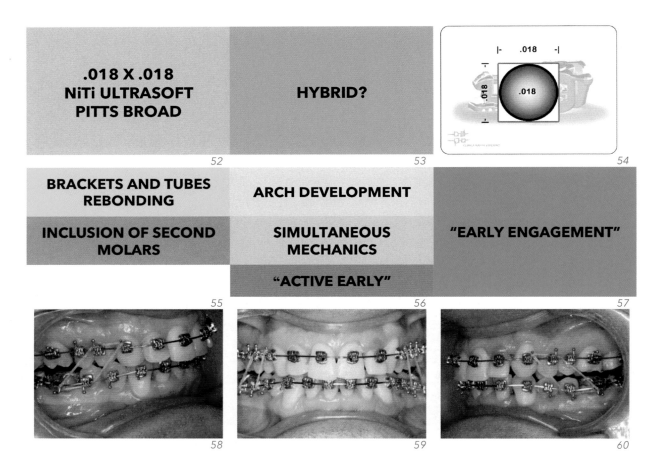

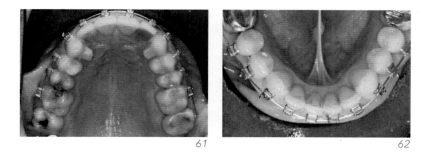

Figs. 63 to 65 We observe that tooth # 22, in which the restorative dentist was going to place a new dental crown (positive coronoplasty), had cut away part of the gum.

Figs 66, 67, and 68 show images of upper and lower .020 x .020" **Niti Pitts Broad** archwires with 3/16" 4 oz elastics.

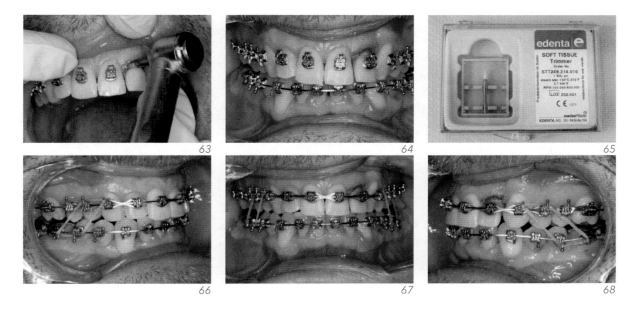

Later, micro-aesthetic detailing is performed to refine the white-pink aesthetic, by decreasing black small angles to gingival of the contact point.

Interproximal reduction is performed to migrate the contact points to the apex.

The closure of those small gaps with a power chain underneath the wire, which, in this case was .020 x .020" Beta Titanium archwire. *Figs 69 to 83*

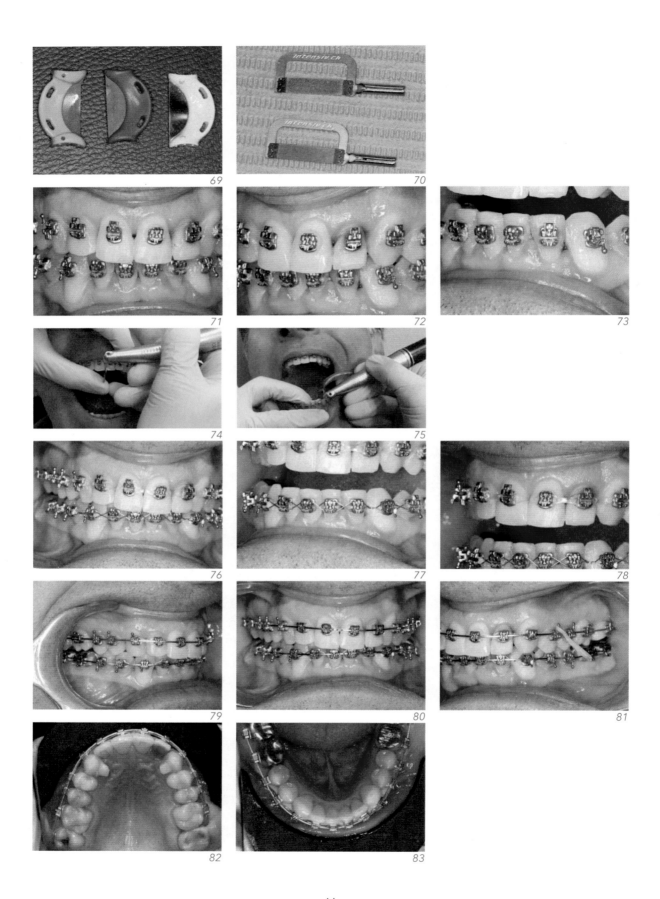

The final details are made using a more flexible archwire, .018 x .018 NiTi Ultra Soft with elastics placed in **L** - 5/16" (diameter) - 2.5 oz (force), and in lateral, between teeth # 24 and 36, 3/16" (diameter) - 4 oz (force) elastics. *(Figs. 84 to 86)*

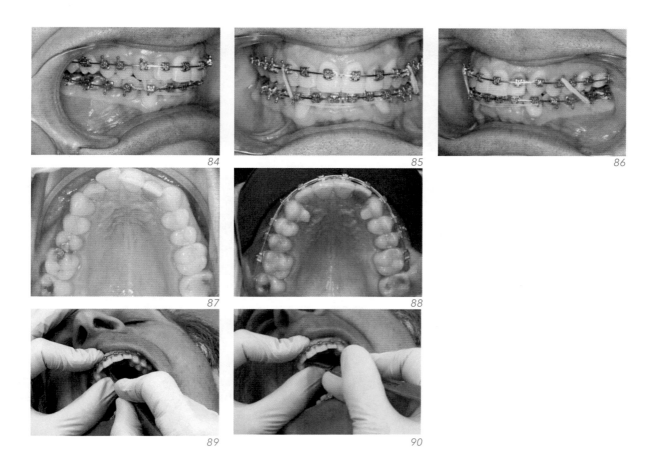

Figures 87, 88, 89, and 90 on the one hand, show the development of the upper arch, and on the other hand a Circumferential supracrestal fiberotomy on the proximal and palatal surfaces of teeth #12 and 22, so that when reinserted in the corrected position we have greater post-treatment stability.

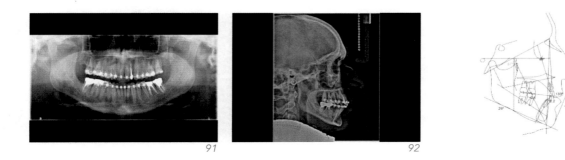

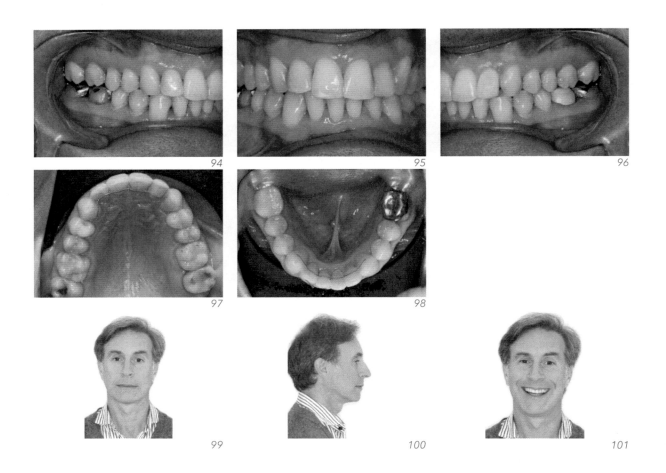

Figures 91 to 101 show the final X-rays, intraoral and facial images, while in *figures 102, 103, and 104* we see that the upper incisor inclinations, which was correct in the pre-treatment **(green)**, is well preserved, as well as a slight clockwise rotation of the occlusal plane.

In the pre and post treatment photographs of the smile, there is a notable improvement in the "buccal corridors", the vertical exposure of the upper incisors (VIP) and the smile arc (SAP). *Figs. 105 to 109*

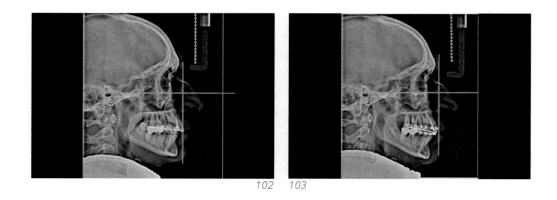

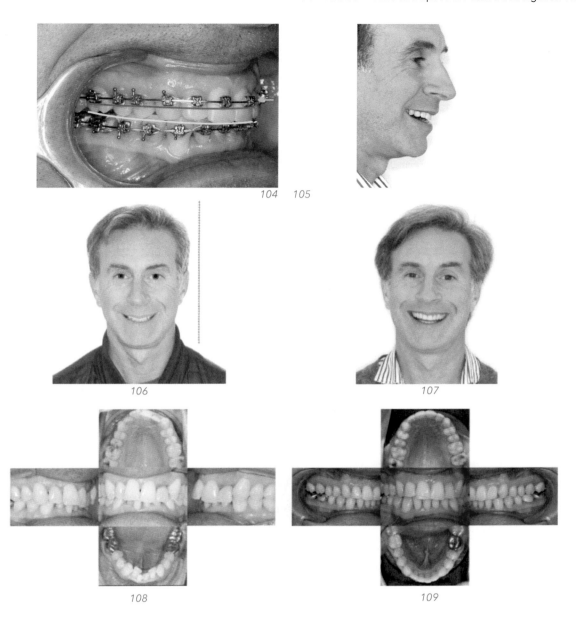

104   105

106

107

108

109

SECTION 2
STAGES IN
SIMULTANEOUS
BIOMECHANICS

Section 2
Stages in Simultaneous Biomechanics
Chapter 4
Introduction

"My favorite things in life don't cost any money. It's really clear that the most precious resource we all have is time..."
Steve Jobs 1955-2011
Outstanding American computer scientist and entrepreneur, founder of Apple.

In orthodontics, treatments were traditionally sequential; the order was transversal problems first, then vertical ones, and later, anteroposterior problems; even in passive self-ligating, the elastics were only used in the steel archwire stage, from posts «crimped» in them.

On the other hand, if there was a muscular imbalance, it was probably approached after treatment during muscle reeducation, with the assistance of speech therapy (logopedia); this entire process can be effective, that is, in leading to the resolution of the case, but it takes a time, which often discourages the patient, especially if the patient is an adult.

At one-point, **Dr. Thomas Pitts** and the excellent collaborator and diffuser of his «orthodontic philosophy», **Dr. Duncan Brown**, began working with simultaneous biomechanics and elastics from the very beginning of the treatments, taking the first big step that was complemented with passive self-ligating brackets with reduced slot, the disarticulation and neuromuscular exercise that leads us to effective and also more efficient orthodontics. *(Figs. 1 to 11)*

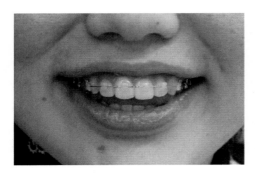

1

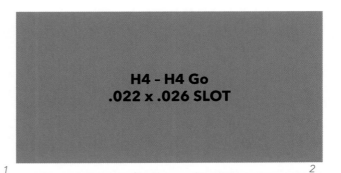

H4 - H4 Go
.022 x .026 SLOT

2

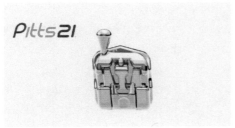

3

PITTS21

.021 X .021 ANTERIOR

.021 X .023 BICUSPID

.021 X .024 MOLAR

4

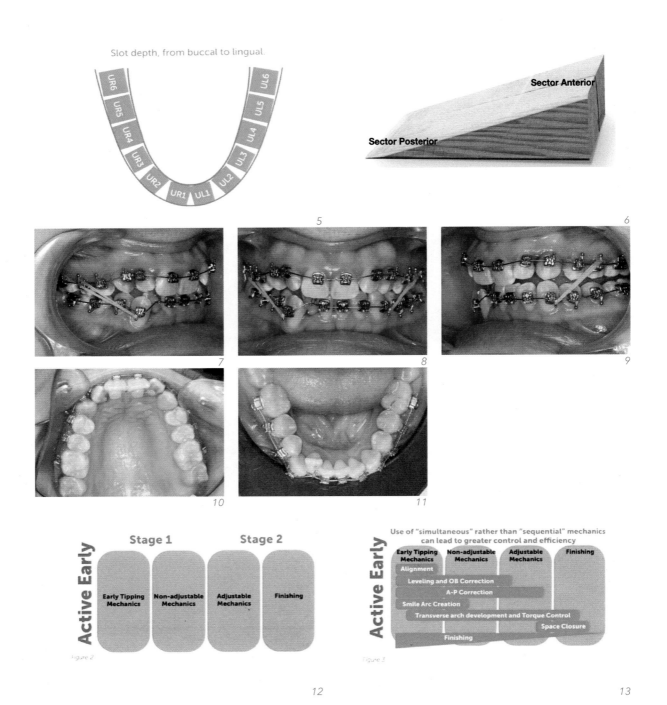

Slot depth, from buccal to lingual.

Sector Anterior

Sector Posterior

5

6

7

8

9

10

11

Stage 1   Stage 2

Active Early

Early Tipping Mechanics   Non-adjustable Mechanics   Adjustable Mechanics   Finishing

Figure 2

Use of "simultaneous" rather than "sequential" mechanics can lead to greater control and efficiency

Active Early

Early Tipping Mechanics   Non-adjustable Mechanics   Adjustable Mechanics   Finishing

Alignment

Leveling and OB Correction

A-P Correction

Smile Arc Creation

Transverse arch development and Torque Control

Space Closure

Finishing

Figure 3

12

13

Following these **«Active early»** multitasking protocols and achieving early 3D control of the teeth with a combination of square slots and square archwires, the **«Early engagement»**, we have noticeable reduced the time-duration of active treatments, obtaining even greater stability in the results.

The order of appointments and what is done in each may vary from one professional to another, but those of us who exhort and attest to the philosophy of Dr. Thomas Pitts, know the value and importance of simultaneous biomechanics to reduce the number of visits of the patient, and this leads to a reduction in number of treatment times.

At our clinic, treatments begin with three appointments very close in time to each other, but different from each other. They are:

1° appointment

Assembly of appliances in the upper arch (generally up to first molars).
Prescription - By choice. (See lecture "Before bonding... Let's think about the prescription" in the ESPARTA Formation platform, _espartaformacion.learnworlds.com_)
.014" NiTi Broad Pitts archwire or .018 x .018 NiTi Ultra Soft Pitts Broad archwire (cases of small dental discrepancy)

2° appointment

Disarticulation + bonding lower tubes and brackets (generally up to first molars)
Prescription - By choice. (See lecture "Before bonding... Let's think about the prescription" in the ESPARTA Formation platform, _espartaformacion.learnworlds.com_)

3° appointment

Goals: Motivation and teaching the use of elastics as well as neuromuscular exercises.

Pursuant to our concept, here is the moment where treatment really begins with the aforementioned Simultaneous Biomechanics **(«Active Early»)**, which saves between 6 to 12 appointments per case, and consequently, the same in treatment time, changing the professional efficiency in a substantial way.

What does the «Active Early» approach involve?

1) Re-contouring of enamel, prior to bonding.
Said negative coronoplasties are smoothed, generally performed in upper canines and without affecting their canine guidance in laterality. Small irregularities in the incisal edges of the incisors, if any, are also softened. _(Figs. 14 and 15)_

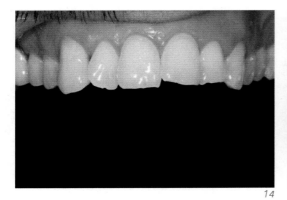 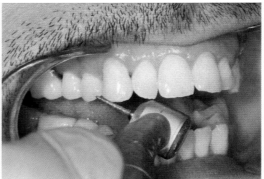

14   15

2) According to Diagnosis **D** there may be reverse procedures to the anterior section, that is to say, positive coronoplasties, adding restorative material in teeth with fractures or excessive wear. Gingivectomies may also be performed.

As far as we are concerned, the gingivectomy that involves a repositioning of brackets, is generally carried out when we bond second molar tubes and advance to .018 x .018" NiTi Ultra Soft Broad Pitts archwires. *(Figs. 16 and 18).*

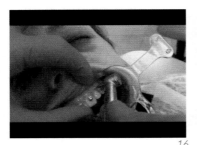
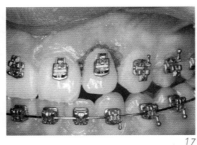
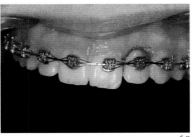

16   17   18

3) Carry out the bonding of tubes and brackets keeping "the final result in mind", this with the aim of achieving both a functional occlusion as well as a good aesthetic, taking as reference mainly the smile arc protection (SAP) the vertical incisor display (VID) and the vertical incisor position (VIP) of the upper incisors.

Remember that with the bonding references in the upper teeth *(see chapter 2 and 3),* the arrangement of brackets, hence the archwire, is not parallel to the occlusal plane (Straight Wire references) but slightly divergent towards the anterior sector (Wedge effect). *(Figs. 19 to 26)*

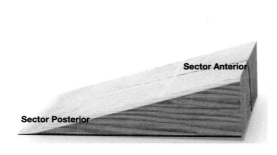

Sector Anterior

Sector Posterior

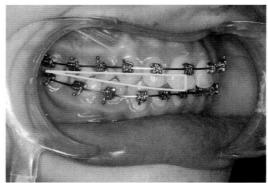

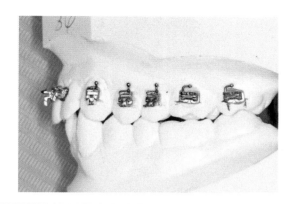

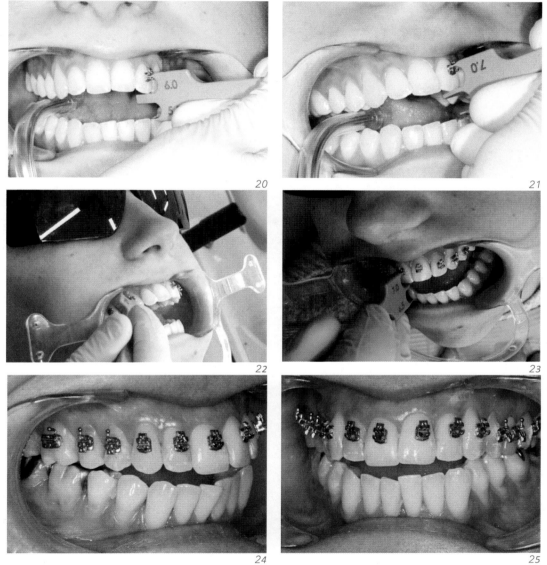

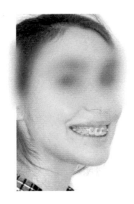

26

1) Bonding the lower teeth according to the requirements of the case and in coordination with what was done in the upper placement. *(Figs 27 a 29)*

Take into account that the bonding of upper brackets is to improve aesthetics and the lower brackets is to improve overbite. Overbite and open bite require differential bonding.

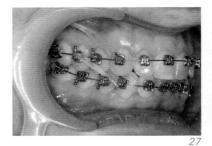
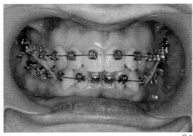
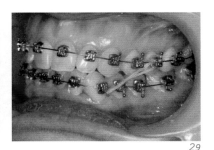

27　　　　*28*　　　　*29*

1) Development of the arches in diameter and perimeter according to Diagnosis **D** and Planning **P**. In our approach, this objective is fulfilled mainly with the use of soft forces released in combination of:

Passive ligation + NiTi archwires; .014" NiTi and .018 x .018" NiTi Ultra Soft Pitts Broad.
Under certain circumstances, said development of the dental arch is enhanced by elastics "through" the arch. *(Figs. 30 to 65)*

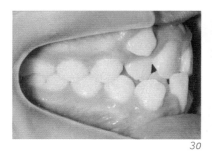
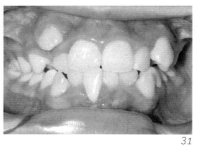
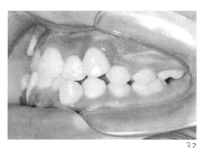

30　　　　*31*　　　　*32*

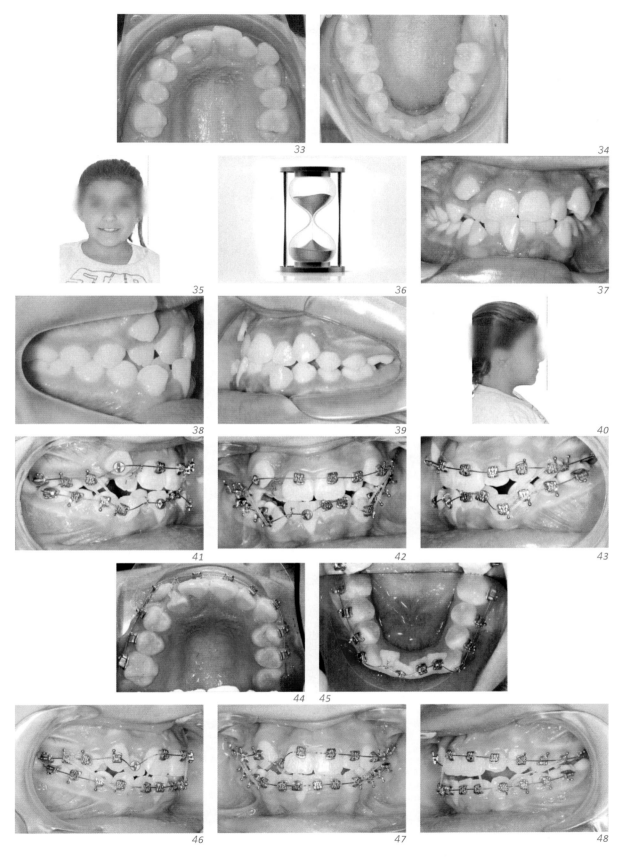

33

34

35

36

37

38

39

40

41

42

43

44 45

46

47

48

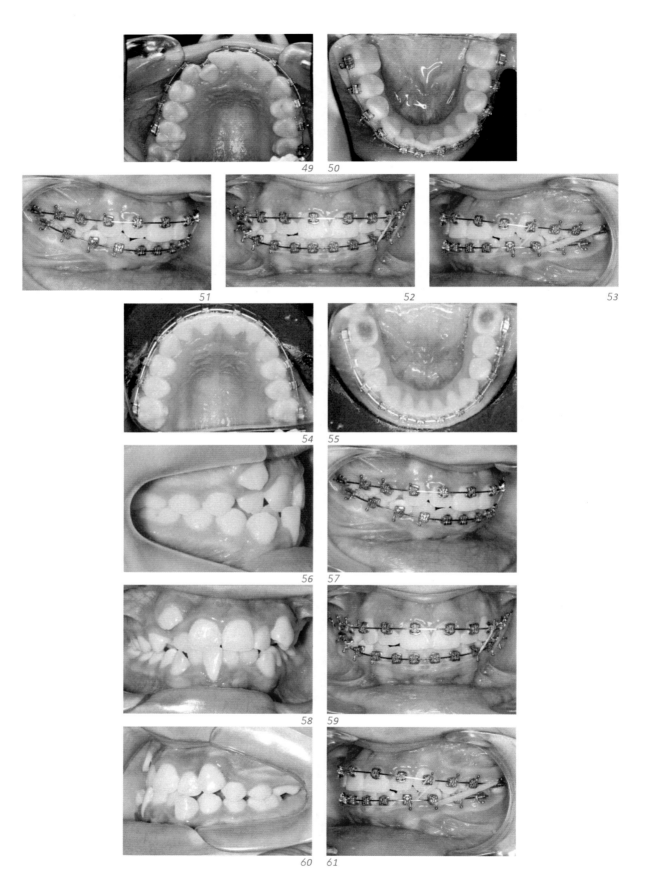

49 50

51 52 53

54 55

56 57

58 59

60 61

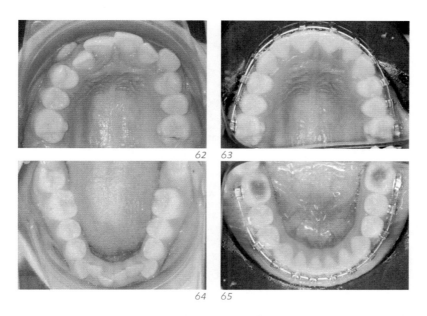

62 63

64 65

PLENITUD LABIAL / TEJIDO BLANDO MENTÓN

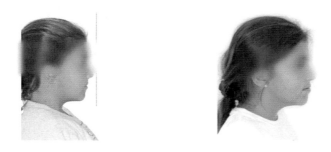

2) Put the triad to work

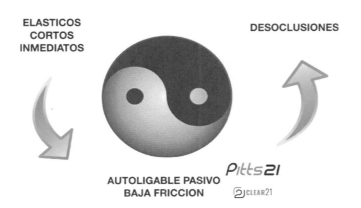

ELASTICOS CORTOS INMEDIATOS

DESOCLUSIONES

AUTOLIGABLE PASIVO BAJA FRICCION *Pitts21* ⓟCLEAR21

These 3 vehicle components **V** are used according to diagnostic needs **D** and with certain biomechanics **B** they depend on and enhance each other.

Orthodontic treatments seek tooth movement to a suitable position through mechanical forces to the teeth. Elastics are a source of force and are used as active components. *(Fig. 66)*

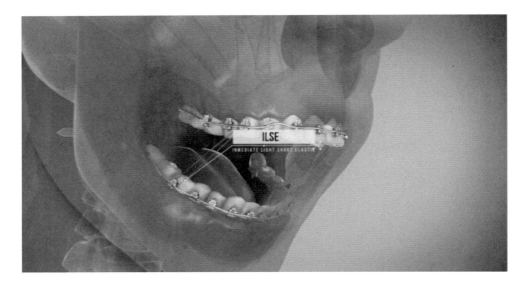

Elastics (ILSE)

- They are more effective and efficient with passive self-ligating systems and associated with disarticulation.

- It's better to use them early, at the beginning of the treatment, rather than later.

- At the beginning and with archwires with a low load-deflection ratio, Light elastics (2.5 oz.) are better.

- At the beginning and with archwires with a low load-deflection ratio, short elastics are better than long elastics.

- They can be used in individual teeth or in groups.

- Must be changed daily. (After 2 hours, elastic strength decreases by 30%, after 3 hours, 40%; Hixon, E. Percentage of elastic force lost in the mouth, Am Jour Orthod. 1970)

- They are not part of the treatment, they are "THE TREATMENT" when there is an intermaxillary problem to be solved, and therefore, it is recommended to use them almost full time. *(Figs. 67 to 76)*

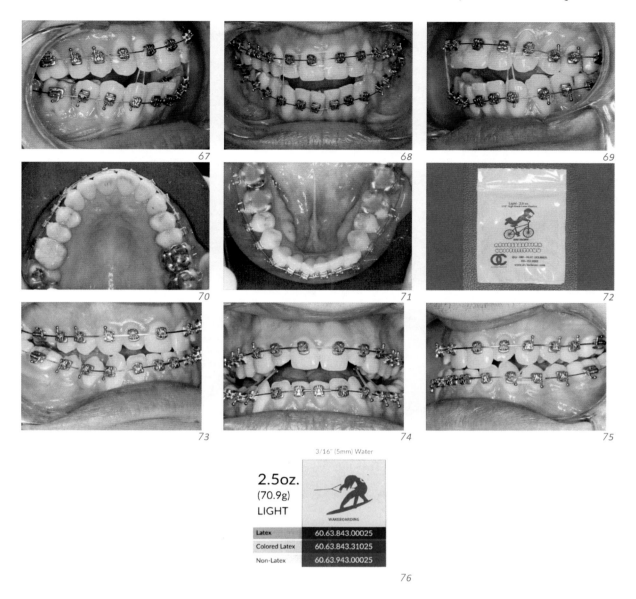

7.   Begin neuromuscular exercise early.

In this section, as a short introduction, we will explain some brief concepts about muscular exercises, which, for certain treatments, we definitely consider it as a fundamental component of the Biomechanics **B**.

There are 3 different types of muscles in the human body, namely:

1) **Cardiac**: obviously present in the heart

2) **Smooth**: in blood vessels, intestinal walls, etc.

3) **Striatum**: The skeletal is the one that is linked to bones and responsible for the displacement or movements that may exist, for example, when walking or running.

Each striatum-skeletal muscle is composed of a vast number of cells or fibers parallel to each other and separated by connective tissue that contains small blood vessels and nerves. *(Fig. 77)*

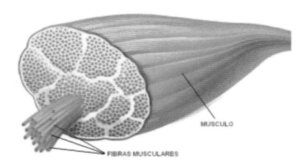

77

- Not all muscles are the same.
- There are stronger and more explosive muscles than others.
- And muscles more resistant to fatigue than others.
- Much of this is determined by the type of fibers in the muscle itself.

There are three varieties of skeletal muscle fibers:

And each type of fiber is unique in its ability to contract in a certain way:

1. **Fast-twitch fibers:**

   Most of the skeletal muscle fibers in the body are called fast-twitch fibers, as they can contract in 0.01 seconds or less after stimulation.
   Muscles dominated by fast fibers produce strong contractions.
   Regarding fatigue, fast fibers wear out quickly.

2. **Slow-twitch fibers:**
   Slow fibers are only half the diameter of fast-twitch fibers and take three times as long to contract after stimulation.
   Slow-twitch fibers are designed so that they can continue working for long periods.

3. Intermediate fibers:

They are a combination of fast-twitch fibers and slow-twitch fibers.

In athletics the physical conformations of a sprinter (100 m), a medium-distance runner (1,500 m), or a marathoner (42 km), are quite different; in the former, fast-twitch fibers predominate, in long-distance runners the supremacy is toward slow-twitch ones, and in mid-distance runners both are combined in fairly similar proportions.

Skeletal muscles, regardless of the variety of the composition of their fibers, can contract in an isotonic or isometric way.

A. Isotonic contraction:

The term "isotonic" means "of equal tension".

In this type of contraction, the fibers of our muscles shorten and lengthen.

Muscle fibers contract and change their length. - Shortening (isotonic concentric): the muscle acts generating tension, to overcome a certain resistance. - Lengthening (eccentric isotonic): before a resistance, we exert tension on the muscle at the same time as we lengthen it.

Certain brachyfacial patients with decreased vertical dimension, masseter muscle contracture, and lower incisor wear may benefit from "3-finger" mouth opening exercises (isotonic eccentric contraction, stretching).

B. Isometric contraction:

"Isometric" means "of equal measure or length".

In this type of contraction, the muscle is static (that is, it neither lengthens nor shortens, its length does not vary, as it does in other types of muscle contraction). In addition, a tension is generated in it. Therapeutically, isometric contraction is widely used for muscle and/or joint rehabilitation as it does not generate stress in the latter; being more "friendly" to them - TM joint.

6. In simultaneous biomechanics in pain patients, we use them to strengthen the elevator muscles, particularly posterior temporal bundles, and as a mechanism of dentoalveolar intrusion in posterior sectors and also in strengthening the TM joint.

8) There are micro-aesthetic procedures already covered in the first section (Patient 2), and they refer to the reduction or solution of "black triangles", gingival to the contact point.

We will simply remember that this situation can be presented by any of these three variables or combinations of them, namely:

1. Triangular or "barrel" shaped incisors.

2. Loss of periodontal bone support before treatment or aggravated during treatment.

3.   Error of parallelism to the axis in bonding brackets.

In certain situations, the complete solution of this problem of micro-aesthetics associated with the white ↔ pink aesthetic relationship requires periodontal surgery. *(Figs. 78 to 88)*

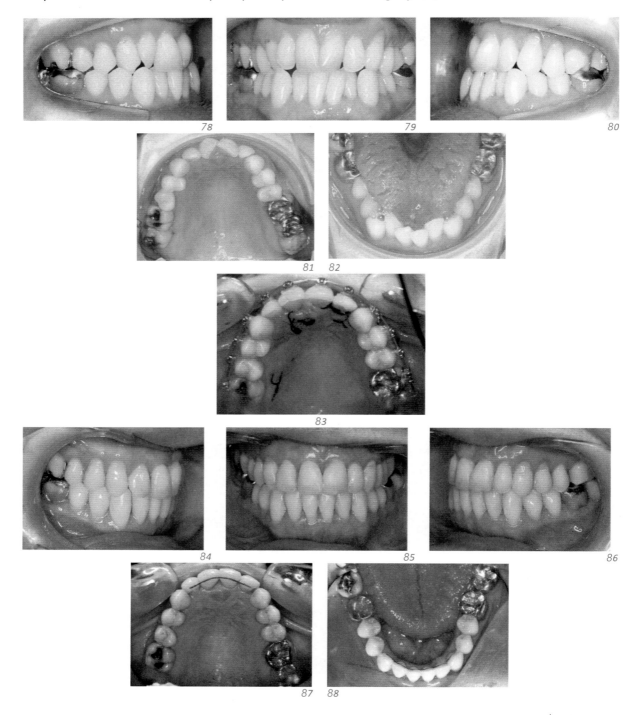

9) Although the results become effective later, the orthodontist should think about the "day after" that is, the active post-treatment containment procedures.

In many situations here, the diagnosis **D** includes retracing the etiopathogenic path of the dysmorphosis that is clinically presented.

In the next chapter of this section, **Dr. Marisa Villalba** will include important concepts referred to in this topic.

Section 2
Stages in Simultaneous Biomechanics
Chapter 5
Patient 3

The trouble is, you think you have time.
Buddha
Siddartha Gautama (563 B.C. – 483 B.C.) Ascetic. Philosopher. (Northwest Ancient India)

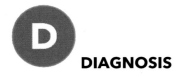

DIAGNOSIS

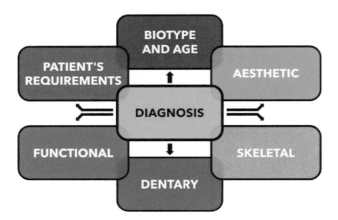

17-year-old patient, mesofacial biotype, with retrusion of the lower third of the face with respect to ideal macro-aesthetic standards.

Poor vertical incisor position (VIP) in the smile of his upper incisors, and lower third of the face decreased in size with respect to the middle third.

Dental area presents:

- Increased overbite, with lower incisal edge reduction.

- Class II.

- Two palatally impacted canine (favorable prognosis)

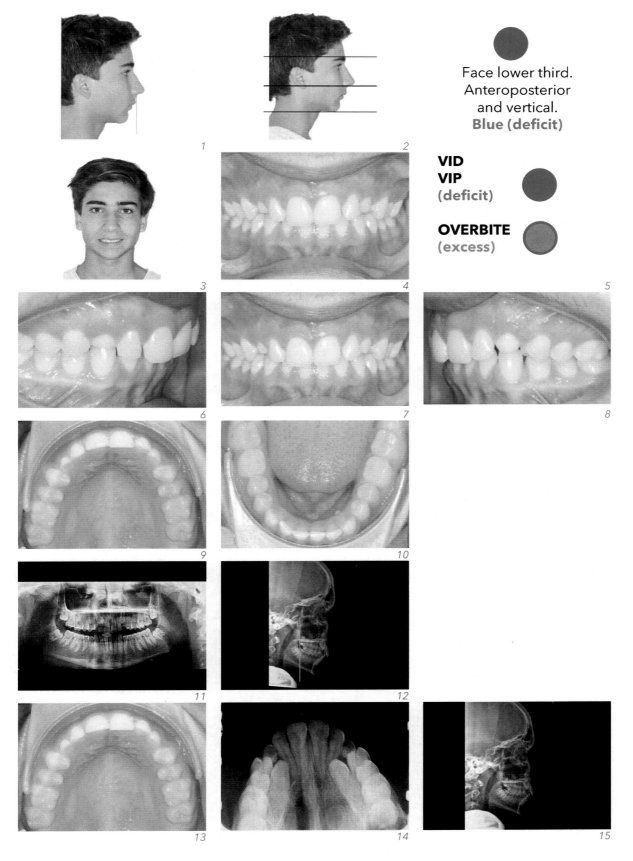

Face lower third.
Anteroposterior
and vertical.
Blue (deficit)

**VID
VIP
(deficit)**

**OVERBITE
(excess)**

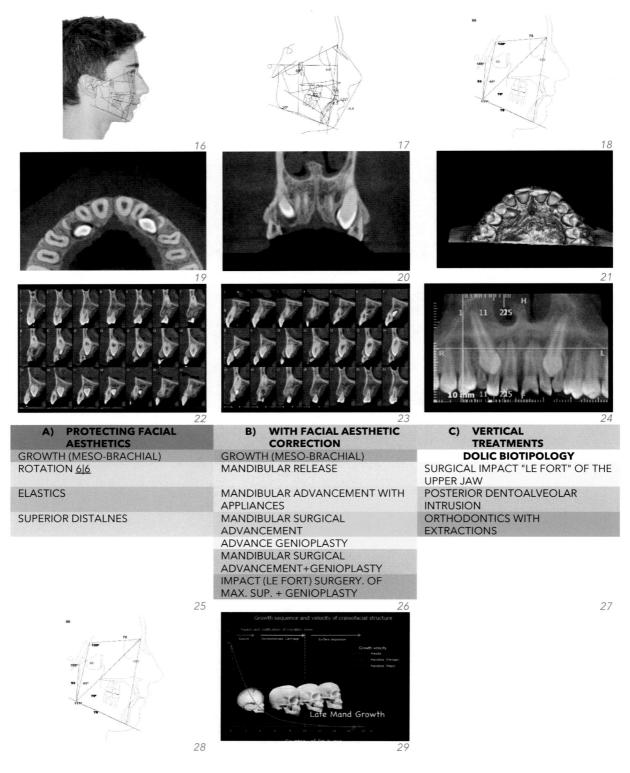

A) PROTECTING FACIAL AESTHETICS	B) WITH FACIAL AESTHETIC CORRECTION	C) VERTICAL TREATMENTS
		DOLIC BIOTIPOLOGY
GROWTH (MESO-BRACHIAL)	GROWTH (MESO-BRACHIAL)	SURGICAL IMPACT "LE FORT" OF THE UPPER JAW
ROTATION 6|6	MANDIBULAR RELEASE	
ELASTICS	MANDIBULAR ADVANCEMENT WITH APPLIANCES	POSTERIOR DENTOALVEOLAR INTRUSION
SUPERIOR DISTALNES	MANDIBULAR SURGICAL ADVANCEMENT	ORTHODONTICS WITH EXTRACTIONS
	ADVANCE GENIOPLASTY	
	MANDIBULAR SURGICAL ADVANCEMENT+GENIOPLASTY	
	IMPACT (LE FORT) SURGERY. OF MAX. SUP. + GENIOPLASTY	

As can be seen in figure 26, our patient is in group B) of our particular classification in Class II treatments.

- Figs. 28 and 29 show two favorable factors for the resolution of class II through the implementation of a treatment that proposes a mandibular advancement, they are:
- Age, remnant growth (17-year-old patient).
- Growth trend (Jarabak).

PLANNING AND THERAPEUTIC VEHICLES (PV)

As there were multiple patient requirements, including aesthetic and intermaxillary corrections, a system of H4 passive self-ligating brackets (PSL) was chosen as the therapeutic vehicle, which was later replaced by Pitts21 in incisors and canines.
Initially, said vehicle was complemented with short 3/16" 2.5 oz elastic and Twin Block-type disarticulations in upper and lower premolars.

BIOMECÁNICA

SIMULTANEOUS BIOMECHANICS	
1.	DEVELOPMENT OF ARCHES (SHAPE)
2.	TORQUE CONTROL (PRESCRIPTION)
3.	UPPER CANINES SPACE
4.	UPPER CANINES SURGERY
5.	UPPER CANINES BIOMECHANICS (TORQUE)
6.	SAP AND VIP DESIGNS
7.	VERTICAL CORRECTION
8.	ANTERO POSTERIOR CORRECTION (CLASS II)
9.	NEUROMUSCULAR EXERCISES
10.	"THINKING ABOUT CONTAINMENT"

Although, we will point out the different stages of the treatment separately, they were approached as Simultaneous Biomechanics, that is to say that these corrections were made together and not sequentially.

CANINE "RESCUE" AND ANTEROSUPERIOR TORQUE CONTROL

- WINDOW surgery, and 45 days-waiting period for self-eruption of said teeth; new gingivectomy and ligation of teeth # 13 and 23 to .014" NiTi Pitts Broad archwire.

- When attaching canines, the NiTi archwire suffers a certain trapping that prevents sliding (Binding), this would generate a protrusion, therefore incisive proinclination.

To control this movement, a 5/16" 2.5 oz elastic (Rainbow) was used; short Class II 3/16" 2.5 oz elastics were also indicated. *(Figs. 31 to 38)*

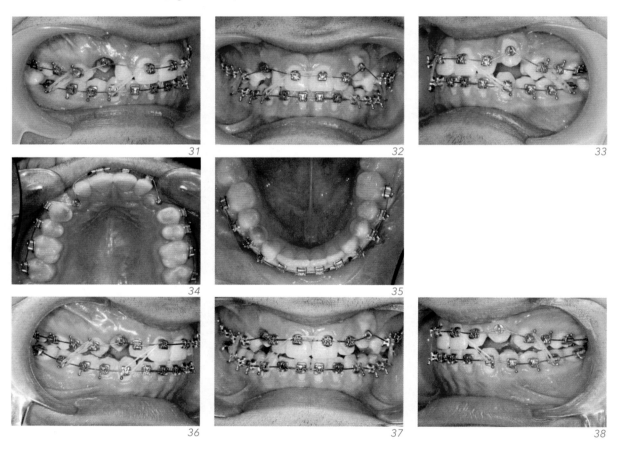

As seen in the images, the disarticulations had been bonded in premolars in the form of Twin Block, resulting in a progressive mandibular advancement proposal. *(Figs. 36 to 38).*

From the beginning, the patient was recommended that he performs neuromuscular exercises consisting of eccentric isotonic contractions (stretching out) of the elevator muscles (especially masseters) with "3-finger" mouth opening exercises. *(Fig. 40)*

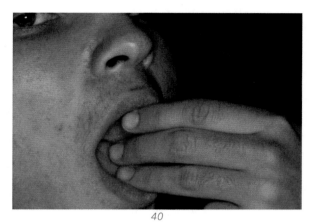

40

We recommend these exercises in 10 daily series of 10 seconds each.

With the inclusion of second molars, we changed to .018 x .018" NiTi Ultrasoft archwires, always combined with elastics and Twin Blocks.

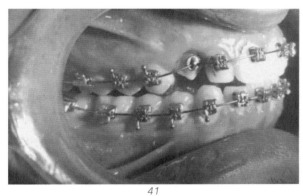

41

Twin blocks were used for 7 months; the last 4 months the mandible must remain in the overcorrection position.

The activation results in an effective progressive mandibular advancement with the addition of material in the mesial slope of the upper blocks.

IT IS CLEAR THAT GROWTH IN THE MESO OR BRACHIAL BIOTYPE IT "ADVANCES" THE JAW, BUT THE BIG QUESTION WILL ARISE:

DOES THE JAW ADVANCE INTRODUCED BY TREATMENT GENERATES STABLE ANATOMICAL CHANGES IN THE A.T.M?

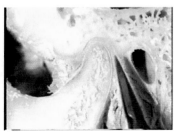

42   43

The gradual mandibular advancement, performed on a "full time" basis, at the growing age, with favorable biotype and structures, make a stable and healthy correction over time possible.

This mandibular advancement would also distend the suprahyoid muscles, apparently contracted, which bring the hyoid to a more posterior position than ideal. *(Fig. 44)*

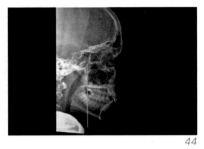

44

When removing the blocks, .020 x .020" NiTi Pitts Broad archwires were installed with short Class II 3/16" 4 oz elastics, and 5 weeks later we continued with .019 x .019 steel wires and biomechanics to close a small gap distal to tooth # 23. *(Figs. 45 to 47)*

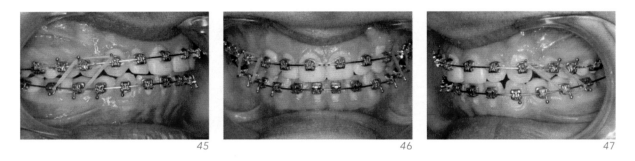

45   46   47

Figures 48 to 69 show final X-rays, and post-treatment photographs of the mouth and face, and video of the patient.

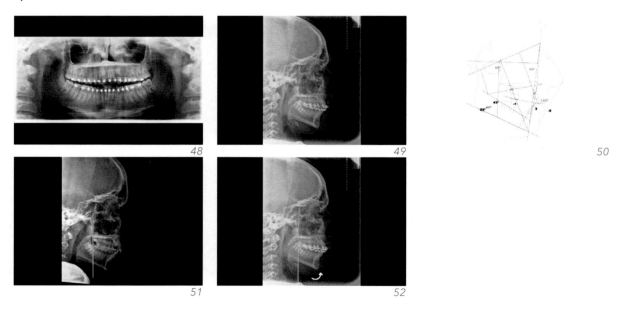

48   49   50

51   52

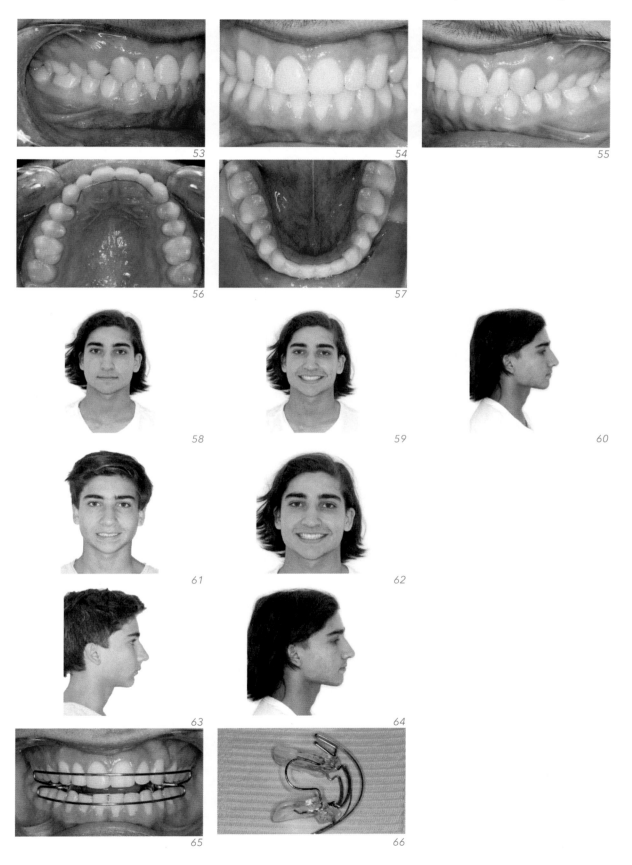

Section 2
Stages in Simultaneous Biomechanics
Chapter 6
Patient 4

"Time passes, as always, it's just a matter of time"
Jorge Wagensberg
Spanish professor, researcher and writer born in Barcelona (1948)

Young adult patient, with dental aesthetic and functional requirements. *(Figs. 1 to 3)*

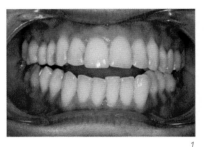
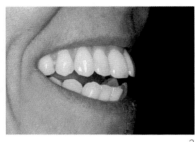
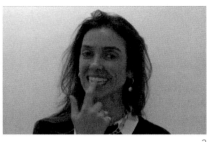

1   2   3

DIAGNOSIS

In **MACROAESTHETICS**:

- Balance of facial thirds **(green)**

In **MINIAESTHETICS**:

- A smile that shows good vertical incisor display (VID) **(green)**

- Reverse curve of smile with SAP absence. **(blue)**

- Excessive incisor proclination. **(red)** *(Figs. 6 to 12)*

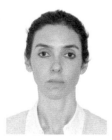
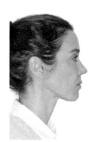
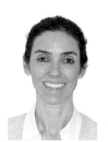

4   5   6

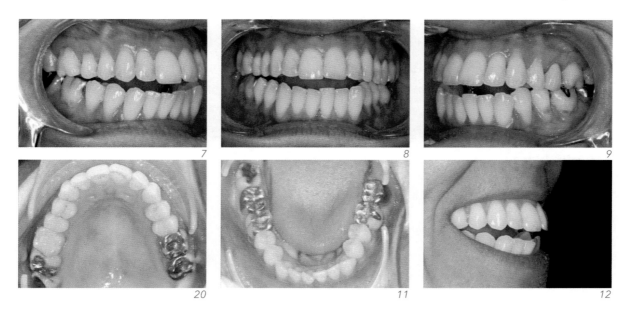

Skeletal/biotypological analysis

Mild Dolichocephalic patient, with open bite and slight basal discrepancy. *(Figs. 13 to 19)*

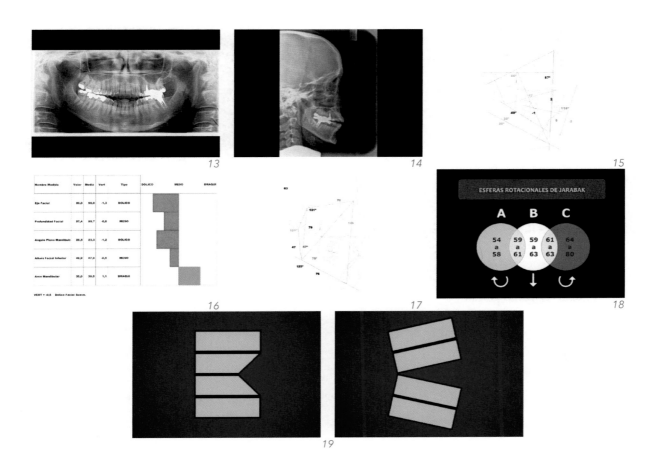

Dental analysis

- The dental area shows an anterior open bite with poor transverse relationship of the arches, a Class I occlusion and -5 mm discrepancy **(blue)** in the lower arch.

- An important aspect of the Diagnosis **D** is that the level of periodontal support was markedly diminished. **(blue)**

- Panoramic X-ray shows several restorations and the presence of 3rd upper and lower molars in the mouth.

- A major swallowing dysfunction led us to question the primary etiology(ies) of this case, which, according to the patient, was mouth breathing and the habit of finger sucking; none of these causes were still active at the beginning of orthodontic treatment. *(Fig. 20)*

PRIMARY ETIOLOGY
• **HABIT/s**
• **ORAL BREATHING**
• **LINGUAL PROBLEMS**
• **DENTAL ANKYLOSIS**
• **GROWTH**

20

PLANNING AND THERAPEUTIC VEHICLES (PV)

Due to the very nice macro aesthetics referred to her profile, the evolution of her nasolabial angle, as well as the critical periodontal problem that she presented:

We are going to start with the **DON'T**

NO PREMOLAR EXTRACTIONS (when the planning objective seeks for anterosuperior retraction, a solution to the negative arch discrepancy in the lower arch, and the anterior open bite).

Then, how is it possible?

To make it possible, planning **WILL** have to include:

1. The development of the dental arches

2. The transverse occlusal relation of dental arches.

3. Extraction of 4 third molars - teeth # 18-28-38, and 48.

4. The antero-superior uprighting, combining the following

    A. The «flocked» (180" turn) prescription in incisors and upper canines. *(Fig. 21)*

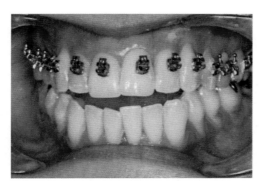

21

    B. Appropriate bonding references, and archwire progressions. *(Figs. 22 to 25)*
    C. Torque, initially in the upper arch, and then in both arches. *(Fig. 26)*
    D. Interproximal reductions (IPR) in upper and lower incisors and canines. *(Figs. 27 to 28)*

5. Posterior dental intrusion to be achieved by exercising appropriate isometric muscle contractions performed on posterior disarticulations.

6. Swallowing re-education with lingual reminders.

7. «Active Early» Protocol for Simultaneous Biomechanics:

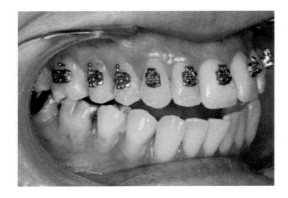

22

.014 TA NiTi Pitts Broad	20x20 BT Pitts Broad	
18x18 TA NiTi Ultrasoft Pitts Broad	Optional 19x19 SS Pitts Broad	SEQUENCE OF ARCHES PITTS21
20x20 TA NiTi Pitts Broad	Optional 20x20 for extra with	

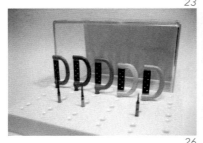

23

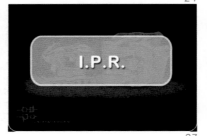

I.P.R.

24

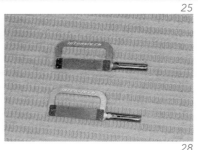

25

26

27

28

THERAPEUTIC VEHICLES (V)

As specified, Pitts21 tubes and brackets were used. The tubes in upper first and second molars have a -27° torque, thus counteracting the proclination generated by broad archwires (Pitts Broad) *(Fig 29-31)*

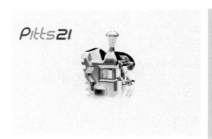

Pitts21

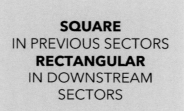

SQUARE
IN PREVIOUS SECTORS
RECTANGULAR
IN DOWNSTREAM
SECTORS

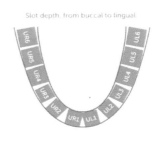

Slot depth, from buccal to lingual

29

30

31

In order to carry out the exercises and muscle re-education, disarticulations were bonded to occlusal surfaces of lower first and second molars, as well as lingual reminders in the lower incisor sector. *(Figs 32 to 33)*

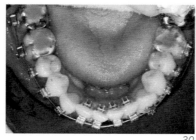

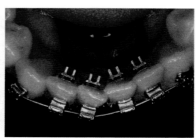

30   31

Also, with adequate Biomechanics , two other vehicles were used to achieve the goals of the treatment plan.

- Pitts Broad Archwires

- Torque Chain

Upon establishing the planning and "vehicles" to be used **P.V**, now we have to move towards an effective and, efficient treatment, approached with «Active Early» protocols of Simultaneous Biomechanics.

B
BIOMECHANICS

1) Started with .014" NiTi Pitts Broad archwires.

2) Lower interproximal reduction (IPR) of 2 mm, 3 to 3.

3) Superior Torque Chain, teeth 14 to 24.

4) Beginning neuromuscular exercising, squeezing in posterior sectors. Quick squeezing 60 times, 6 times a day, was recommended.

5) Bonding lingual reminders to the lower incisors; the squeezing exercises were complemented with lingual support in upper ridges and palatal vault (lingual lifting). The tongue is curious, but not stupid, and flees from reminders by modifying its low positioning.

6) 5/16" light 2.5 oz elastic, linking upper and lower incisive sectors. *(Figs. 34 to 41)*

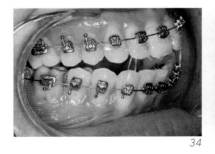
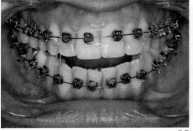
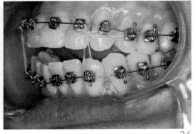

34 *35* *36*

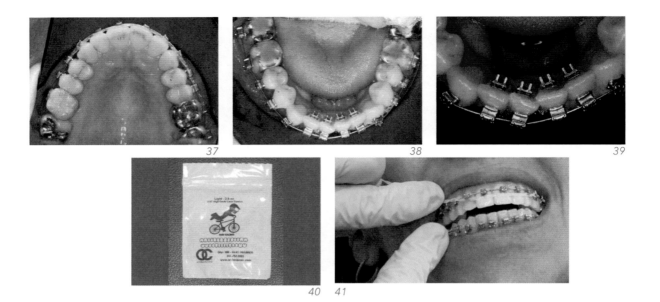

37 38 39

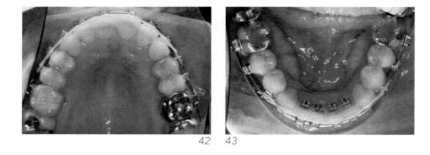

40 41

The second archwire used was .018 x .018" Niti Pitts Broad and the occlusal photographs taken 2 weeks after installation show us a surprising result in rotational correction, thanks to the early engagement with 3D control achieved by the relationship between arc/slot. *(Figs. 42 and 43)*

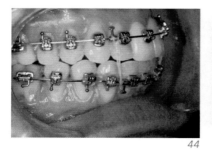
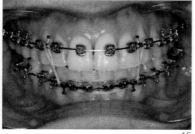

42 43

Archwire progression and Simultaneous Biomechanics continued with .020 x .020" NiTi Pitts Broad archwires, now with «crimped» posts, 5/16" 2.5 oz rainbow elastics.

And the neuromuscular exercising and lower torque chain also continued. *(Figs 44 to 49)*

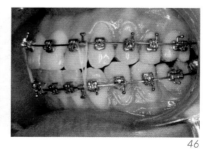

44 45 46

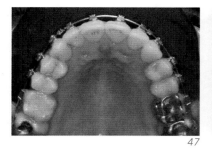
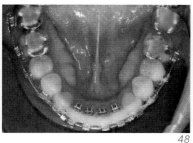
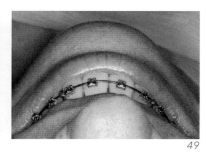

47   48   49

Then, .020 x .020" B titanium archwires were also installed on «crimped» posts.
A small interproximal reduction on mesial surfaces of teeth # 11 and 21, added to the elastic chain below the arch, solved a micro-aesthetic problem (black triangle and contact point to gingival direction, showed in photographs 50 to 52).

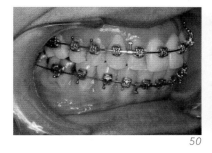
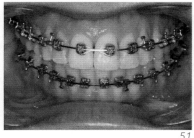
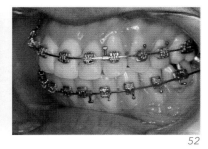

50   51   52

Figures 53 and 54 show the anterior-superior retraction compared to the pre-treatment. *(Figs 55)*

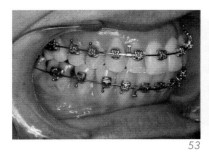
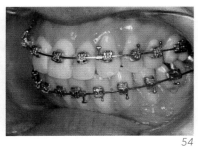
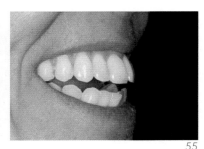

53   54   55

Figures 56 to 68 show final X-rays as well as photographs of the mouth and face.

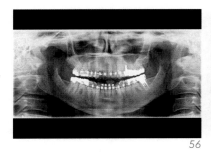
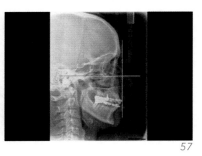
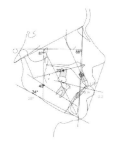

56   57   58

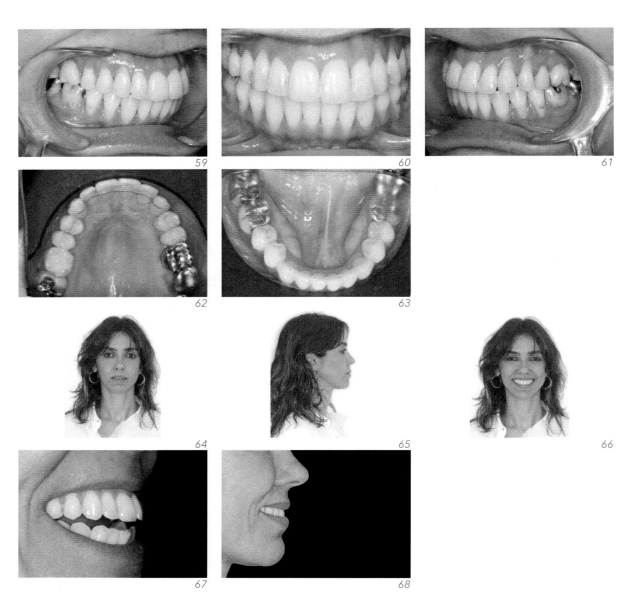

When comparing figures 68 and 69, we observe the change in the upper incisor inclination between pre- and post-treatment (one of the patient's requirements).
Beyond the fixed bonded palatal and lingual retainers between upper and lower canines and incisors, the nightly use of Bionator (Bimaxillary functional appliance) was recommended. *(Fig 69)*

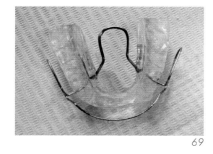

69

Section 2
Stages in Simultaneous Biomechanics
Chapter 7
The Role and Origin of the Dysfunction in Treatments

"I love the external simplicity, which shelters a great internal complexity"
Miguel de Unamuno
Spanish write and philosopher, part of the Generation of '98 (1864-1936)

Introduction

The etiology of the malocclusions that we observe in daily practice have been studied and analyzed by great masters from ancient times to modern day, and it is subject to discussion between different philosophical currents. There are those who believe that the origin of a malocclusion would be subject to inheritance or genetics and there are those who exhort and support the theory that the origin of the malocclusion would be the influence of the epigenetic - environmental on the individual, where the alteration of one or more vital functions, influence the maxillary and mandibular growth and dentoalveolar development, and results in a "deformation" of the system, due to compensation or adaptation to said alteration.

- In these cases, we think about the "FORM-FUNCTION" BINOMIAL. The shape of the maxilla and mandible, and the development of the dental arches will be the result of the balance of muscular forces during vital functions. If the FUNCTION is altered, the "SHAPE" will be altered, while if the FUNCTION is correct, the SHAPE of the maxilla, mandible and dentoalveolar will be correct.

- Undoubtedly, we cannot put "all eggs in the same basket", that is, not all cases can be included within one theory or another, but it is clear that there are concepts and knowledge that we cannot ignore or lose sight of.

- We need to consider the child, teenager or adult patient as a whole, and the dental position should not be the only objective of our treatment. We must bear in mind that a "dysfunction" may be responsible for both the ORIGIN of the malocclusion, as well as the LOSS OF STABILITY after treatment.

In this chapter, we will review briefly which are the FUNCTIONS that we must assess and detect when imbalanced, serving dual purposes according to the orthodontic stage of our patient:

- If it is a growing child, it will be useful to eradicate it in time, and redirect the child's development.

- If our patient is in the post-treatment stage, it will be useful to assess the functions to determine if these factors will give stability over time or if we will have to keep them in mind to reeducate them, and we will not consider the orthodontic treatment "finished" until they are fully rehabilitated, otherwise any gains will be easily forfeit.

- Finally, we will see the THERAPEUTIC possibilities and some of the VEHICLES and MYOFUNCTIONAL EXERCISES that we can use in this rehabilitation to reach the end goal: dental alignments and normal occlusion in a healthy and balanced muscular and functional system, where the muscles themselves maintain the orthodontic gains.

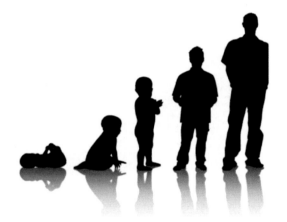

Dental Dysfunction and Occlusion

If a dysfunction is installed early and is not diagnosed or intercepted in time, the child will grow up in this situation and we may later find a teenager / adult with dentoalveolar and skeletal problems.

Our mission will be to keep in mind the concepts of normality to be able to identify when the functions are altered and whether or not they were responsible for the etiology of the malocclusion, taking this into account to rehabilitate the patient before or during orthodontic treatment.

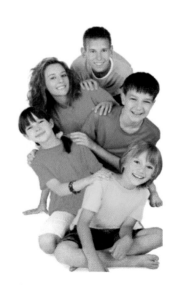

What is causing the problem?

Let's not just stare at the "surface"; what we can see with the naked eye, the misaligned teeth are a SIGN/SYMPTOM of the problem, NOT the problem itself; we must observe in "depth" the possible dysfunctional factors that would be causing the alteration of the system, to eradicate them and restore balance.

THE GENETIC? or ...
A FUNCTIONAL IMBALANCE?
▪ MOUTH BREATHING
▪ ATYPICAL SWALLOWING
▪ ORAL HABITS
▪ POSTURE
▪ INADEQUATE CHEWING
▪ PSYCHOLOGICAL PROBLEMS

In this "depth", we will have to assess: the facial muscle function, breathing and swallowing mechanism, lingual and body posture, as well as sleep, food, emotions and lastly, analyze the possibility of some existing genetic component that will help us as a guide to know "the soil" where we will work and its possible responses to therapy.

Functional analysis

Shape - Function Binomial

As suggested by Dr. Melvin Moss in his functional matrix theory **"THE FUNCTION MAKES THE SHAPE"**. We have to imagine how the set of facial muscles that surround the dentoalveolar structures are working during activity in vital functions through the shapes we see.

- We should imagine the conformation of dental arches as the result of "struggles" between centripetal forces (from outside to inside) and centrifugal forces (from inside to outside); if muscles work with each other in coordination, we will obtain a "balanced" system, while if any force exceeds its opposite, the "imbalance" or "alteration" will appear in the shape of the area where these forces acted.

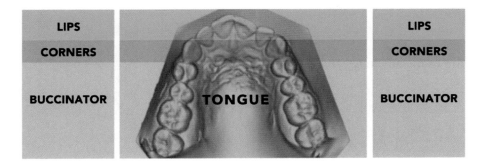

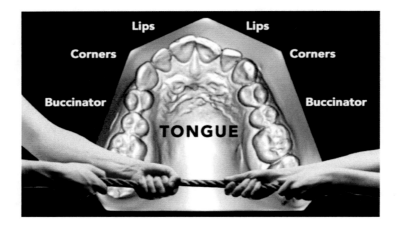

Let's analyze each muscle individually.

The tongue.

The tongue will exert its shaping action both at rest (tongue positioning) and during function. Knowing that this organ is formed by 17 muscles is of utmost importance, since it is considered a great shaper of the adjacent structures. If its position is correct at rest and its behavior is balanced in function, the "shape" of the arches, maxilla and mandible will be optimal both in the dentoalveolar development stage and in post-treatment containment.

A. TONGUE POSITIONING

It is the resting position of the tongue within the oral cavity. The normal and correct position will be:

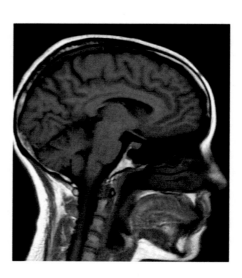

- Tongue tip in palatal ridges

- The dorsal sector that follows the tip is barely separated from the bone palate, generating a space called a "bubble".

- The rest of the back of the tongue is in contact with the hard palate and soft palate.

- Laterally, it is in contact with the palatal and lingual surfaces of the molars.

B. LOW TONGUE POSITION

- It is the alteration of the normal resting position.

- For different reasons it is in a lowered position, causing alterations at the dentoalveolar and skeletal level that we will see later.

- The important thing here is to know how to identify when the tongue is "low" in the child, teenager or adult, to correct the habit before or after orthodontic treatment and achieve stability over time.

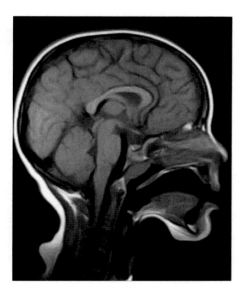

- The simplest and most practical way to evaluate the resting position of the tongue is by observing the position of the hyoid bone in the lateral skull teleradiography: tracing the "HYOID TRIANGLE" at plain sight or by means of a drawing on the teleradiography. The hyoid triangle is made up of the following:

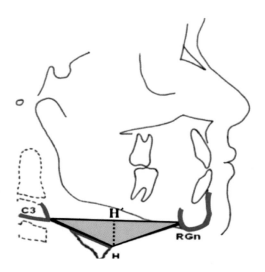

Cephalometric points:

C3: most anteroinferior part of the 3rd cervical vertebra.
RGn: most posteroinferior point of symphysis.
H: "hyodale" most anterosuperior point of the hyoid
H": perpendicular projection to C3 - RGn plane.

- The connection of these 3 points form a triangle with an upper base and a lower vertex, where the distance from "H" must be up to 5 mm from H".

- When the tongue at rest is **LOW**, the arrangement of the triangle is modified. The triangle becomes a "line" or an "inverted triangle" by varying the position of the hyoid.

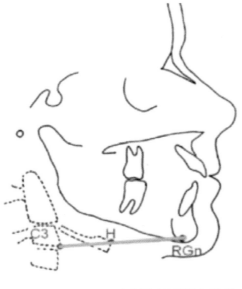
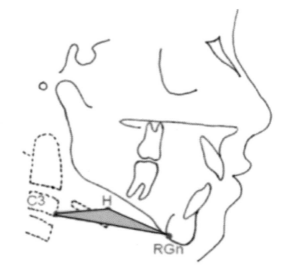

LINEAR TRIAGLE   INVERTED TRIANGLE

Some manifestations and clinical signs of a possible low tongue:

MAXILLARY NARROWNESS

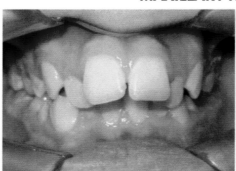
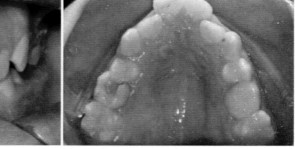

SHORT FRENULUM, TONGUE-TIE

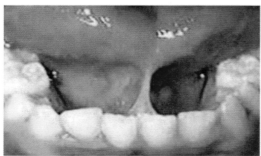
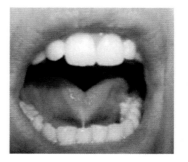

TONGUE PLACEMENT AGAINST OR BETWEEN TEETH

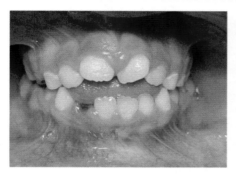 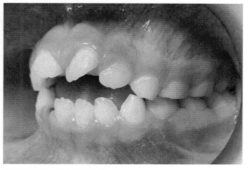

DEEPER PALATE IN THE MAXILLA

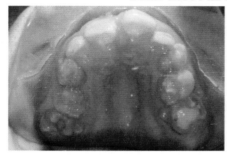 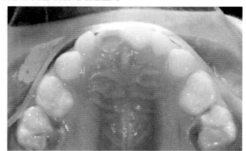

- When we identify a low tongue in the patient, we have different therapeutic possibilities to rehabilitate it, either during the functional orthopedic treatment in the case of children, or undergoing low friction orthodontic treatment when patients are adults.

- In the case of functional orthopedic appliances, most have a lingual reminder or positioner called "Coffin", a rigid 1.2 mm "U" wire located in the palate that the patient must touch with the back of their tongue, to strengthen the muscles of the same tongue and train where it must rest.

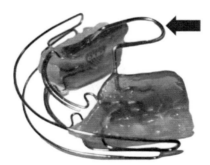

- Another very effective therapeutic vehicle in myofunctional therapy to achieve the repositioning of the tongue is the MYOBRACE (MCR) trademark system and THE TRAINER SYSTEM, which consists of various designs according to the patient's needs and age, to achieve the main objective of functional rehabilitation.

- Within this system these are the specific devices for lingual training, and other devices will have specific accessories to lift and reposition the tongue, as well as other accessories for the rest of the oral muscles.

MYOBRACE - Lingua line

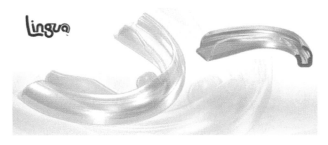

It is placed only in the upper jaw and has a tongue tab that serves as a reference for the correct tongue position, which in turn forces the patient to breathe through the nose. It can be used day and night.

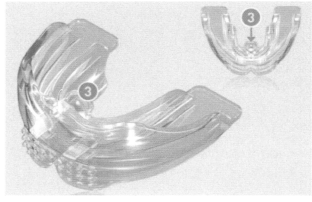

There is great variety within the MYOBRACE system depending on the age of the patient.
They all have in common this "tab" which is a tongue "positioner" par excellence.

- Within the MYOTAELA line of MYOBRACE, we can use the TLP (Tongue and Lip Press) and the TLJ, which is useful not only in rehabilitating the tongue, but also the lips.

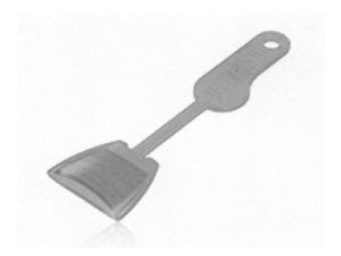

Active myofunctional appliance aimed at the tongue and lips that need greater strengthening and additional tone to obtain stable results in orthodontics.
Lack of muscle strength/tone can also be a contributing factor in increasing the risk of breathing disorders during sleep.

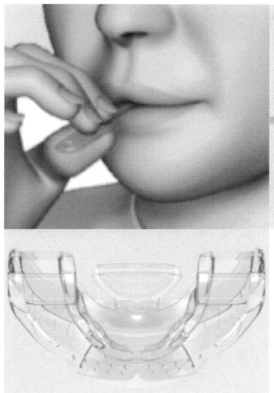

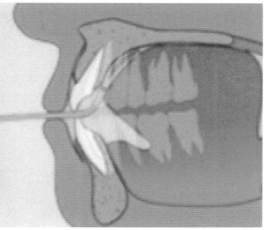

The tongue of the device will provide muscle strength or tone to the tongue and rehabilitate its position.

- In the case of a teenager or adult with low friction orthodontics, we also have "lingual reminders", which will be of great help so that the patient can rehabilitate the tongue and correct its low position, while performing orthodontic treatment.

- They are metallic attachments that are located on the lingual surface of lower incisors, a place where the hypotonic and dysfunctional tongue usually rests. These reminders will cause such discomfort that the patient must have to lift the tongue to the correct place.

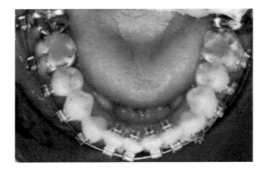

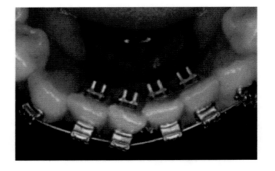

- There are also a series of exercises (see myofunctional exercises section) in our philosophy with the Dr. Pitts bracket that we can suggest to our orthodontic patient to perform during treatment, that help lingual training.

- One of them is the "lingual lifting" exercises as a reference of where to position the tip of the tongue. It consists of asking the patient to place a piece of chewing gum on his tongue and lift it against the palate with enough force to "crush it" in the area of the palatal ridges.

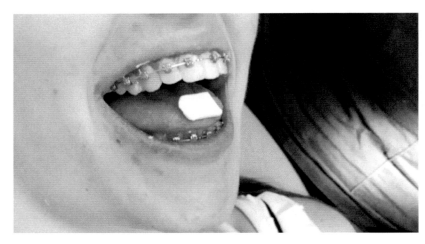

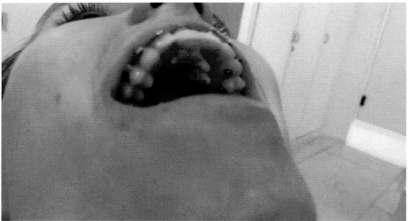

- In conclusion, it is very important to evaluate from the beginning both the position and the lingual function of the patient, at any age, and if an anomaly is detected, it will be resolved as soon as possible by choosing the most suitable therapeutic means for it.

Lips

The lips, represented mainly in their anatomical constitution by the orbicularis oris muscle, have the function of providing competence to the oral cavity in chewing, swallowing and resting.

- The lips also participate in phono-articulation, in changes in facial expression that facilitate unspoken language and have great aesthetic importance in the affective part. They also give sensitive information about the foods that will enter the mouth. To carry out their multiple functions, the lips require an associated muscular support system.

- The perioral musculature is made up of the following fascicles:

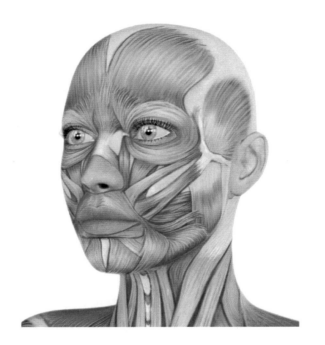

- Buccinator muscle

- Canine muscle

- Mentalis

- Orbicularis oris muscle

- Depressor labii inferioris muscle

- Triangularis

- The lips fulfill their "MODELER" action in 2 situations:

FUNCTIONS	Swallowing	Breathing	Phonation
HABITS	Lip Suction		

- In **FUNCTION**, they must achieve an effortless bilabial closure, that is, that the closure is carried out at the expense of the simultaneous contraction of the orbicularis muscles, both superior and inferior. When, bilabial closure is not possible due to a lack of tone in any of them, the nature "compensates" for this situation, since in order to swallow it will be necessary to create a negative pressure in the oral cavity; So, if the orbicular muscles do not have enough tone, other muscles will perform the contraction, and the alterations of the bilabial closure will appear, with consequences related to the affected area.

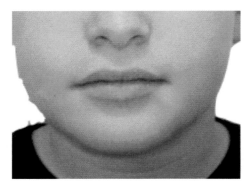 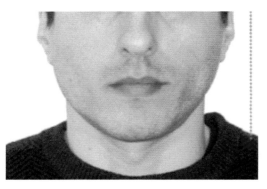

- In **HABITS**, lip interposition or suction is one of the causes that generate greater "deformation" in the dentomaxillary system of the anterior sector. Placing the lower lip against the palatal surface of upper incisors, and suctioning it, will break the anterior dental guide, creating the so-called "lip trap", which, when sustained over time, will further deepen the distance between upper and lower incisors.

- The immediate consequences will be:

  - Proclination of upper incisors

  - Retroinclination of lower incisors

  - Overjet/overbite increase

- At the mucosal level, this habit is easily detected by irritation of the mucosa and perilabial skin.

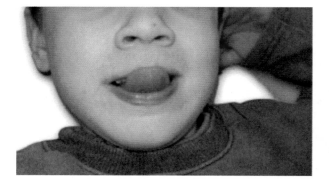 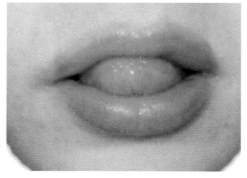

Lip Closure Alterations

· LIP WITH TOOTH

In this alteration, the anterior oral seal is at the expense of the lower lip in contact with the palatal surface of the upper incisors. There is the presence of a "lip trap", which is the space left by the lower lip when it is placed between the incisors. The proclination of the upper incisors observed on clinical inspection was generated by the presence of the lower lip, at rest and in function.

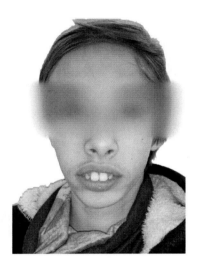
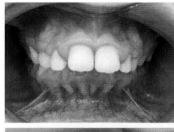
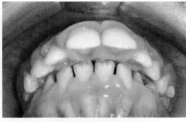
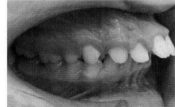
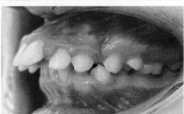

· CLOSURE EFFORT

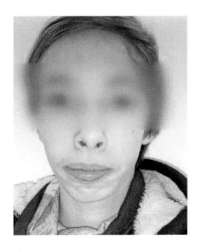

Due to lack of tonicity in the orbicularis oris muscle to achieve anterior hermetic closure and to be able to start swallowing, the most common alteration to observe is hypercontraction of the mentalis muscle, clinically visualized as a dotted or "orange peel" in the chin area. If we observe this situation, we must be careful to assess the presence of a muscle dysfunction and its consequences.

- In the following example, we also observe the altered bilabial closure, where lip with tooth and closure effort due to the hypercontraction of the mentalis are combined when the swallowing begins, revealing the dysfunction.

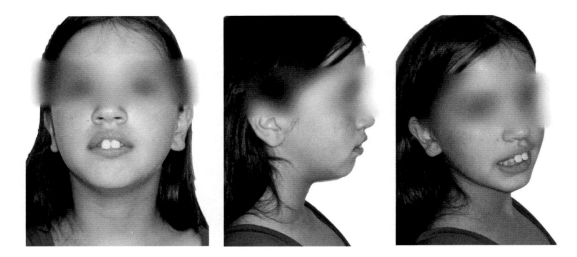

- The dental consequences of this dysfunction will be evident when going to the clinical examination:

  - Proclination of upper incisors

  - Retroinclination of lower incisors

  - Narrowness of the maxilla

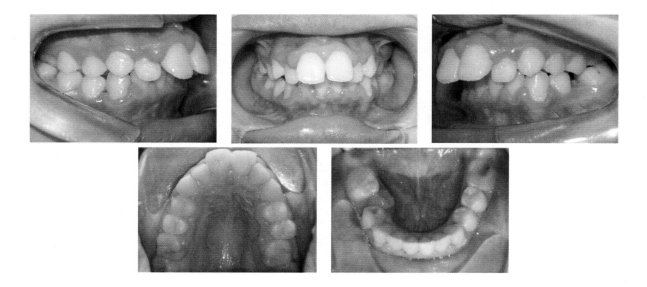

- This is where we should take a few minutes and think "who" was "responsible" for this oral disorder before deciding on the treatment or of therapeutic vehicle.

- The dental proclination shows to be the product of the interposition of the lower lip between the teeth and the depth in the maxilla is due to the low tongue.

- The resolution of the case is very simple and surely, we will not be wrong; We will only have to decide which is the indicated therapeutic vehicle to remove the poorly positioned muscles and correct them, both with functional and orthodontic appliances.

In the case of a completed orthodontic treatment, I consider that part of the decision to grant the final discharge to our patient will be to confirm that the patient is normalized and muscularly and functionally balanced.

Regarding the lips, we have to verify that the bilabial closure at rest and in function, is "effortless", and just with the tone of the lips, without involving the rest of the muscles of the perioral area. Thus, we will have a **balanced system**.

Lip and lingual trainers.

Within the myofunctional therapies, we have specific devices to rehabilitate muscle functions. Some may be manufactured with their own elements according to the skill and creativity of the professional; and others we may acquire directly from a particular trademark; For example, the "MYOBRACE" system has a line called MYOTAELA that includes:

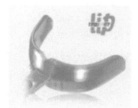  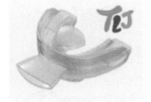 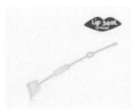

1. **LIP TRAINER:** it is designed to be used with other appliances to improve lip seal, increasing the tonism in the orbicularis and decreasing the hyperactivity of the mentalis (which is activated in atypical swallowing). It is used 2 times a day for 5 minutes and overnight, to sleep.

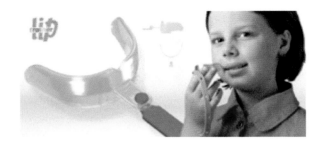

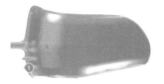

Lip bumpers: deactivate the strong muscles of the chin area

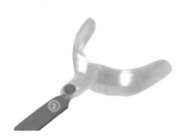

Safety band: exercises the labial muscles

2. TLP: "tongue and lips press": it is designed to train the muscles of the lips and tongue that require greater strength and tonicity to obtain orthodontic stability in our treatments. We can indicate it while the patient is undergoing orthodontics, since its use is external and does not prevent the correct development of the arch. The system brings a series of exercises to perform.

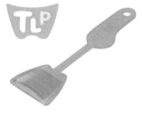

Indicated for mouth breathers and atypical swallowing patterns where there are low tongues and lack of lip seal

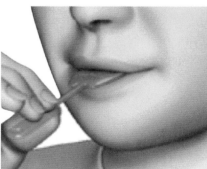

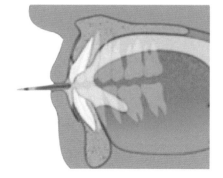

3. TLJ: "Tongue, Lips and Jaw": it is indicated for patients who present muscles without strength or tone in the lips, tongue and problems in the TM joint. Each part of this appliance is designed to train these muscles through exercises to be performed by the patient.

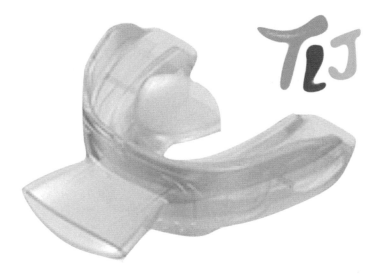

4. LIP SEAL: works on lip tonicity and sealing. It is indicated in mouth breathing patients with lack of strength and incorrect lip posture at rest.

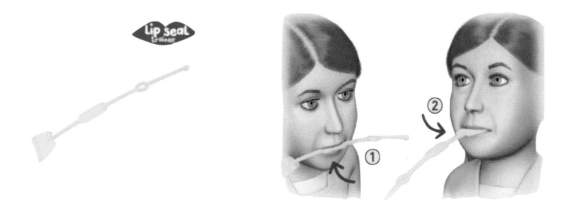

Sub-section:

At the end of this chapter, there is a description of a series of exercises for the patients that can be performed both with commercial appliances and also using the creativity of the professional with elements that meet the same objective: to rehabilitate lip function.

Breathing.

- Normal and physiological breathing must be NASAL. The nose is designed by nature in order to filter germs and particles from the air that enter from the external environment.

- Then the nasal conchae will have the function of stopping that flow of air that enters, to favor the mixture of oxygen with nitric oxide. This gas is produced by the paranasal sinuses when breathing through the nose, and has very important vaso-dilating properties that will favor the absorption of oxygen at the lung level.

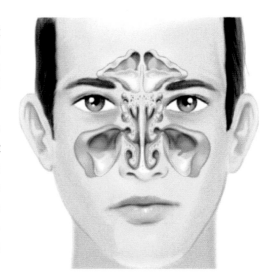

- The paranasal sinuses also have the function of heating and warming the cold air that enters from the external environment to reach the lungs with the closest temperature and humidity to the internal environment (37° and 44mg / l).

- During nasal breathing, it is necessary for the mouth to be closed at some point. This is usually by the lip sealing. But this closure can also occur in the middle portion of the tongue in contact with the hard palate and also later with the base of the tongue against the soft palate.

OUR DEFENSE SYSTEM: WALDEYER'S RING

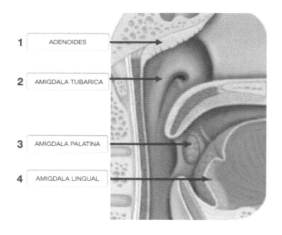

1 ADENOIDES

2 AMIGDALA TUBARICA

3 AMIGDALA PALATINA

4 AMIGDALA LINGUAL

- Physiologically, the lymphatic tissue is part of our immune system, a system that will recognize between what is proper to the body and what is not; and identifies it and attempts to remove it. Waldeyer's Ring is one of the lymphatic tissues formed by 4 structures located around the naso and oropharynx, the entry point to the upper digestive-air tract.

- This ring represents between 3% and 5% of the lymphoid tissue and is of great importance in the respiratory process, since the hypertrophy of 2 or more of its structures can greatly alter the nasal respiratory function.

1. PALATINE TONSIL

- They are commonly called "tonsils" and are located in the oropharynx between the palatoglossus and palatopharyngeal muscles and are closely related to the soft palate, tongue and oral cavity. They are an important defense barrier, generating IgA and IgE that are defense factors against bacterial or viral microbial agents.

- They are active between 4 and 10 years and then regress. Hypertrophy or excessive growth due to permanent functioning can generate different degrees of oropharyngeal obstruction.

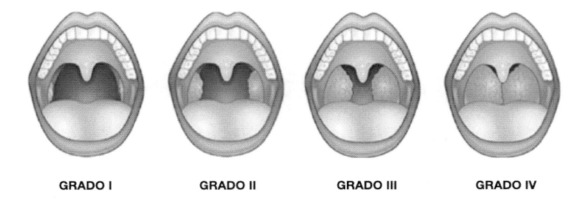

GRADO I   GRADO II   GRADO III   GRADO IV

- Clinical image of hypertrophied tonsils. This can be diagnosed clinically at plain sight when the patient opens his mouth.

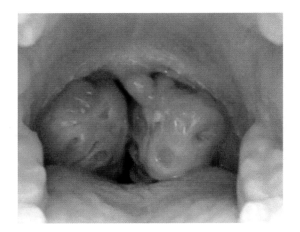

- They grow when the nose does NOT work.

- When hypertrophied they have no defense function.

- Breathing, swallowing and apnea problems

2. ADENOIDS

- They are an accumulation of lymphoid tissue located in the upper back part of the pharynx, between the nose and throat.

- These, unlike the tonsils, are not seen clinically. Its inspection can be done through lateral skull teleradiography.

- The function of the adenoids is to filter germs and particles that enter through the nose, producing antibodies against infections. If these occur repeatedly, the adenoids grow or hypertrophy causing respiratory problems due to the impossibility of the passage of air, an issue that must be resolved as soon as it is diagnosed, since the patient by survival instincts will breathe through the mouth when he cannot breathe through the nose, and this action will have consequences that we will see later.

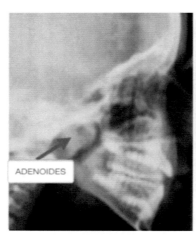

ADENOIDES

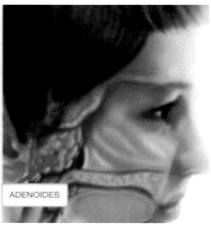

ADENOIDES

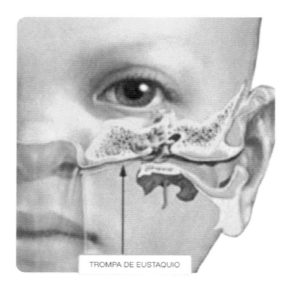

TROMPA DE EUSTAQUIO

Adenoids and ear infection

The adenoids in turn, due to their proximity to the Eustachian Tube (runs between your middle ear and pharynx), will cause repeated ear infections or otitis because of the permanent bacterial presence that will reach the middle ear through the Eustachian Tube.

3. LINGUAL TONSILS

They are located at the base of the tongue. They are a non-encapsulated lymphatic aggregate of a variety of sizes.

4. TUBAL TONSILS

They are located in the tubal fossa, in the lateral wall of the pharynx and connect the nasopharynx to the middle ear. From the 4 lymphoid structures, the **palatine tonsils** and adenoids are the best known and the ones that commonly complicate the respiratory process.
The degree of hypertrophy and the final decision of removal will be subject to the otorhinolaryngologist decision, but we, as oral health professionals, must not fail to identify them as a possible cause of respiratory disorders, with their dentomaxillary consequences.

Mouth Breathing.

The knowledge of the disadvantages of altered physiological breathing is of historical date; there are evidence and scientific studies that support and describe the complications caused by mouth breathing.

| 1855 - 1930 | 1920 - 2003 | 1927 - 2014 | 1936 - 2018 |

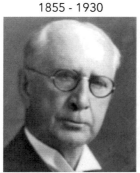 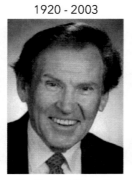 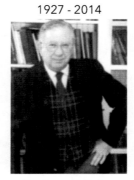 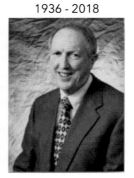

Dr. Edward Angle *Dr. Robert Ricketts* *Dr. Donald Enlow* *Dr. William Proffit*

"The cornerstone of facial growth is the nasal breathing." The face grows around the airways: if these are working properly, the face develops forward and clearly defined. On the contrary, if the airways do not function properly, hypoplastic facial and jaw development will be lacking.
Dr. Donald Enlow
"The harmony in the position of the teeth, the size and relationship of the arches is influenced by another force, the muscular pressure; of all the causes of malocclusion, mouth breathing is the most frequent in all ages."
Dr. Edward Angle

"The respiratory function has been the most overlooked factor in clinical orthodontics. In the 30s and 40s, the "phenetic" concept dominated in skeletal alteration, leading to treating only the teeth rather than the face or the patient as a whole. The information on the "failures" of that time, highlights the respiratory problems as influential.
Dr. Robert Ricketts

"The factor in dental balance is the pressure exerted by the tongue and lips at rest. Breathing influences, the posture of the head, jaw and tongue, therefore if breathing is disturbed, the balance is broken."
Dr. William Proffit

- Breathing is the MOST IMPORTANT VITAL FUNCTION, not only because it allows us to survive, but also because the rest of the functions depend on it for their normal develop. **It is the cornerstone**. If breathing is altered, that is, mouth breathing instead of nasal breathing, there is no possibility that swallowing, chewing and phonation will develop normally.

- When there are difficulties in nasal breathing, there is a substitution for mouth breathing. There are patients who breathe through the mouth with no apparent cause other than a bad HABIT. But in general, the most frequent causes of mouth breathing are OBSTRUCTIONS or FLACCIDITY of the perioral muscles.

The Obstructions can be:

- Hypertrophy of adenoids

- Septum deviation

- Foreign body

- Hyperplasia of the mucosa

- Tumors

- Polyps

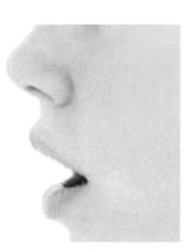

- Mucosal hyperplasia can be caused by: allergic rhinitis, sinusitis, irritation due to odors or pollution.

- Pharyngeal hypertrophy occurs due to hyperplasia of the palatine tonsils

- The hypo-tonicity of some muscles of the face can also generate the constant mouth opening, and so the patient breathes through the mouth.

FACIAL CHARACTERISTICS

- Collapsed and immobile nostrils
- Flat cheekbones
- Dry and flaky lips
- Dark circles
- Tired face

DENTAL CHARACTERISTICS

- Narrow upper arch
- Low tongue
- Small and retruded maxillary base

  Increased incidence of cavities

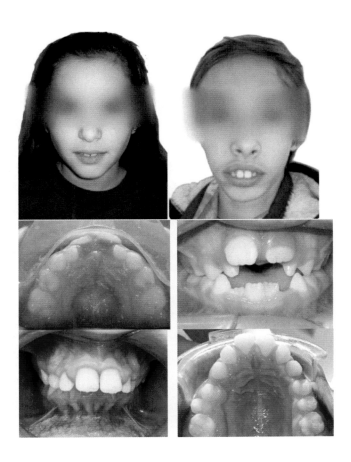

POSTURAL CHARACTERISTICS

When the patient needs to open his mouth to breathe in, he needs to change the position of his head, shoulders and spine so as not to lose his balance and fall forward. That is why there is a series of "accommodations" of the body to stay being upright and balanced.

- Forward head
- Cervical spine in hyperextension
- Forward shoulders
- Dorsal spine - Kyphosis
- "Bourgeois" belly
- Lumbar spine - Lordosis

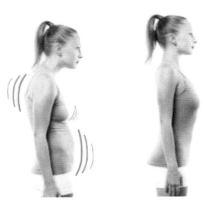

NEW LINGUAL POSITION

- Tongue in most anterior position
- Parted lips
- "Hanging" mandible by relaxation of elevators
- Decreased activity of nostrils dilators
- Bad rest, does not deepen sleep

RESPIRATORY DISORDERS OF THE MOUTH BREATHER

- Amigdalitis
- Hipertrofia Adenoides
- Sleep apneas
- Tonsillitis
- Adenoid hypertrophy

TONSILLITIS

- They grow when the nose does NOT work
- When hypertrophied, they have no defense function
- Swallowing, breathing and apnea problems

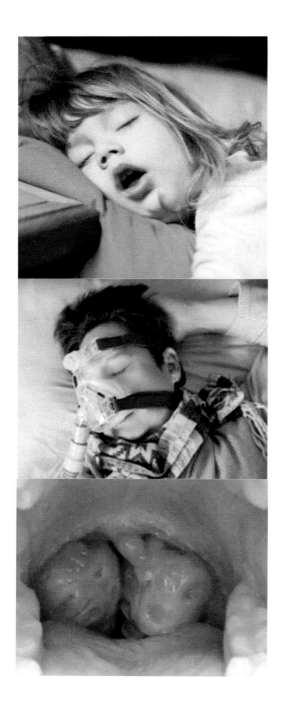

Therefore, it is essential to search for the cause of the mouth breathing and not just to assess the symptom. Nature is wise: if air does not enter through the nose, it will enter through the mouth in order to survive. This modification of the position of the mouth causes the whole system to adopt another position as well, and in these attempts to "compensate", the system begins to fail.

MOUTH BREATHING AND SLEEP

The new lingual position in the mouth breather and the sleep disturbances is something that we cannot lose sight of. SLEEP is a biological activity that we must take care of as it is the moment where the entire system has the physiological capacity to regenerate and repair. If the child or adult "sleeps badly", the consequences will be seen during the day. And sleeping "well" has to do mainly with having a physiological "nasal" breathing where the oxygen that reaches the lungs enters purified, humidified and tempered. If the patient sleeps with his mouth open, and is still growing, the secretion of the most important development hormone, Somatotropin or GH, will be affected. This hormone is released after 2 or 3 hours of deep sleep, when the child is in stage 4 or NON-REM sleep. This deep stage is reached if the patient can fall asleep with normal breathing. If the patient breathes through the mouth, there are micro-awakenings and he will not reach stage 4.

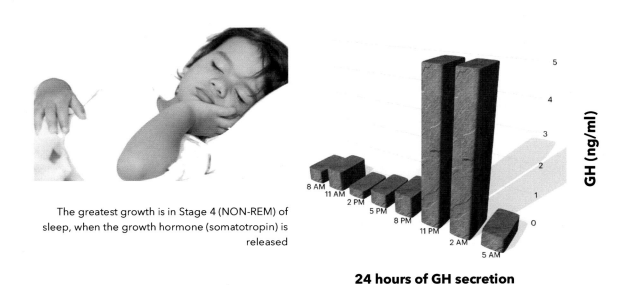

The greatest growth is in Stage 4 (NON-REM) of sleep, when the growth hormone (somatotropin) is released

24 hours of GH secretion

Another consequence of sleeping with the mouth open is the lack of stimulus for transverse development of the maxilla due to the absence of the tongue on the roof of the mouth.

- An adult who breathes through his mouth at night will also have issues: sleep disturbances (micro-awakenings, snoring, hypopnea or sleep apnea) that will later bring him problems in his daily life, since he will be a poorly rested and oxygenated person. He may suffer from drowsiness, general tiredness, and lack of concentration on his tasks. At the dental level, he will have the same consequences as the child.

ASSESSMENT OF THE MOUTH BREATHER

The assessment will be in detail. When we have a possible mouth breather, we must not forget that this dysfunction affects several anatomical structures directly, and others indirectly in a form of a "cascade effect"; thus, we will find a postural imbalance as well as a dysfunction in chewing, swallowing and even phonation.

In a first appointment, we must create a warm environment, where the patient feels comfortable and safe. The first diagnostic tool will be the ANAMNESIS AND simultaneously the observation of the spontaneous BODY POSTURE. We will observe how is the position of the head and posture of the body in relation to his shoulders, from

the frontal and profile view, standing and sitting, while we are talking with him, without making him feel observed, so he is not conditioned to adopt a posture, instead, the posture is the most natural possible.

ANAMNESIS

We will ask the patient or his parents a series of very simple questions about daily moments.

While your child is sitting (watching TV)

- Does he put things in his mouth? (toys, sleeves, pencils, nails, etc.)

- Does he suck his lips?

- Is his mouth open, even just a little bit?

- Is his tongue between his teeth?

- Does he make noise when breathing?

- Does he have a hard time being still?

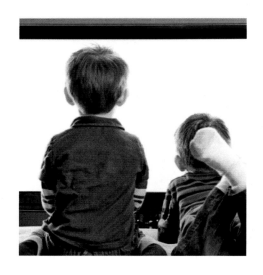

While your child talks

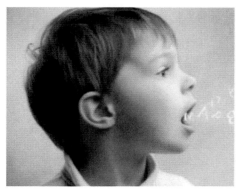

- Does he speak too fast?
- Does he speak too slowly?
- Does he stop to breathe?
- Does he have a lisp?

While your child eats

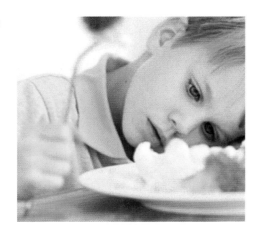

- Does he stop breathing between bites?
- Does his tongue stick out when he swallows or drinks?
- Does he make noise when he chews?
- Does he eat sloppily?
- Does he take a breath when he drinks?
- Are his lips tight when swallowing?
- Does his chin wrinkle when he swallows?
- Does he tilt his head when he swallows?
- Does he have difficulty being still?

While your child sleeps

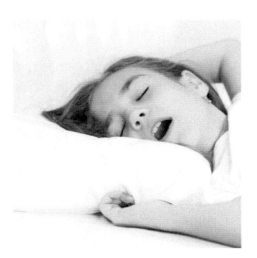

- Is his mouth open?
- Does he snore?
- Does he wet the bed?
- Does he toss and turn?
- Does he wake up frequently?
- Does he have nightmares?
- Does he grind his teeth?
- Does he have troubles waking up?
- Does he have dark circles?
- Does he wake drooling or with dry saliva on his face?

While we are carrying out the questionnaire, we must pay attention to some "signs" that can also show evidence of the existence of respiratory problems.

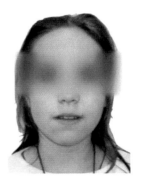

- Dark circles/tired and sad face
- Dull and lost look
- Excessive salivation
- Halitosis
- Tiredness when speaking
- Lack of coordination to breathe and speak simultaneously

ASSESSMENT OF THE RESPIRATORY FUNCTION

There are several simple tests to perform in our office both, in children and adults. Here we will mention one of the simplest tests: the ROSENTHAL test, which serves to differentiate whether mouth breathing is organic or due to some anatomical alteration. Before the test, it is necessary to verify that the patient is not undergoing any acute inflammatory process (cold, allergy, etc.)
It consists of 3 steps:

1. The patient is instructed to keep his mouth closed until we notify him. We count 20 full breaths as we observe the chest movements he performs. He must not notice this so that he does not alter the rhythm.

2. We insist that he continues with his mouth closed, and request him to occlude the right nostril with his right thumb. We return to observe the thoracic movement in 20 breaths.

3. We ask him to continue with his mouth closed and now he will occlude the left nostril with the left thumb and we count the 20 breaths again, observing the respiratory movements. Here the test ends.

Test conclusions:

- If the patient achieved 60 breaths, first with both nostrils and then one at a time, and did not increase his respiratory rate or open his mouth to enter the air, we have a patient with good air passage.

- If there is an anatomical obstruction, his breathing rate will increase until he opens his mouth, no matter how much he wants to comply with the given command.

In this case, our responsibility will be to refer the patient to an ENT consultation to be diagnosed and treated on time.

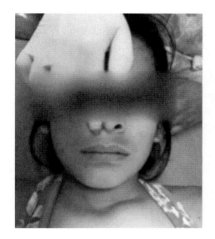 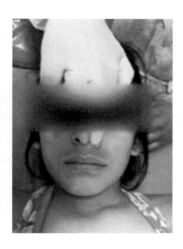

Clinical Case

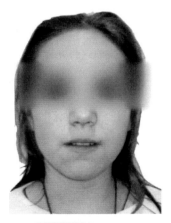

In the facial analysis, in the frontal view we observed: dark circles, flattened malars, hypotonic collapsed nostrils, parted lips without contact, dryness and a fatigue face look.

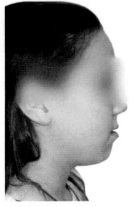

In the facial analysis, from the profile view, we observed the same characteristics described, adding the hypo-development of the maxilla and the pathognomonic sign of a low tongue, which "double chin".

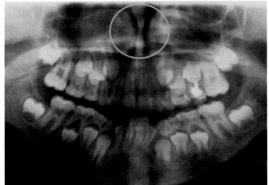

In the panoramic X-ray, a radiopaque area is observed at the level of the nostrils, suggesting the presence of some hypertrophy of the turbinate mucosa or allergy.

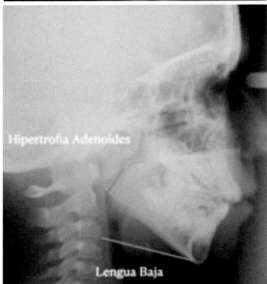

In the lateral teleradiography of the skull, at plain sight, we observed the decrease or narrowing of the lumen of the upper airways (hypertrophied adenoids), and the low position of the tongue. The latter is a conclusion resulting from the tracing of the hyoid triangle with a linear result (and not a triangle with a lower vertex)

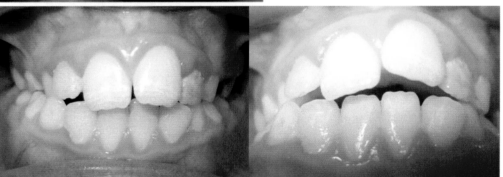

At the oral level, we will find the consequences of dysfunction:

- Narrowed maxilla or ogival palate.
- Dental proclination
- Tooth crowding
- Lack of anterior guidance

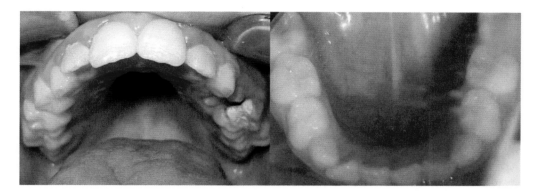

A patient was diagnosed with mouth breathing due to hypertrophy of adenoids and nasal conchae with associated allergies, and was referred to ENT for treatment. Simultaneously, functional orthopedic treatment begins to gradually shape the arches at the expense of the rehabilitation of the position of the tongue, both at rest and in function.
A Klammt Elastic Open Activator (KEOA) is placed.

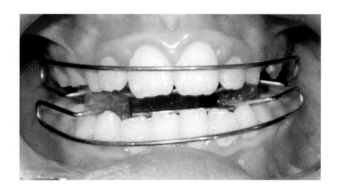

KLAMMT ELASTIC OPEN ACTIVATOR

It is a rigid bimaxillary device that generates isometric forces. It is a regulator of functions, that is, when the device is placed in the mouth, the muscles adopt their correct position and can be reorganized to perform their functions correctly. In conclusion, it will be reorganized and rehabilitated muscular system itself that restores harmony to the dental arches, maxilla and mandible, dental positions and finally the face in growth stages.

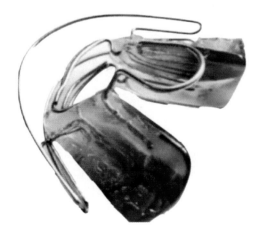

COMPONENTS:

- **Buccal arch**: placed in the buccal third of the teeth, in the anterior sector, it controls the position of the incisors, and in the posterior sector it works as a "barrier" to avoid compression dentoalveolar ridges by the buccinators.

- **Palatal and lingual arches**: they are placed inside on the palatal and lingual surfaces of upper and lower incisors, and together with the buccal arch, they control the anteroposterior position of the incisors. (They are placed in contact or not, as needed).

- **Coffin or transpalatal arch**: it is a reminder par excellence of the normal position of the tongue, both at rest and in function.

- **Acrylic**: it is the connecting element of all the wires described and its function is to determine the working position of the device to generate the isometric forces necessary for rehabilitation.

Intermediate stage of treatment

The forward position observed is the result of the KEOA construction bite, which is worked in 3 space directions with the aim of developing muscular isometric strength; this must be **forward, lowered and centered**.

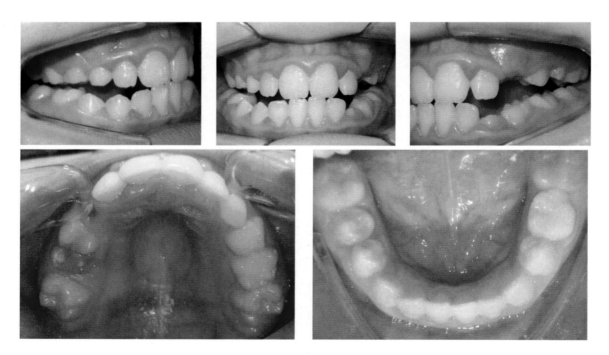

- The patient uses the device for 16 hours daily, and all night to sleep. With this therapeutic vehicle, we will accompany the dental replacement and development of the arches, eliminating those muscular forces that "prevent" the growth in the case of a patient with temporary or mixed dentition.

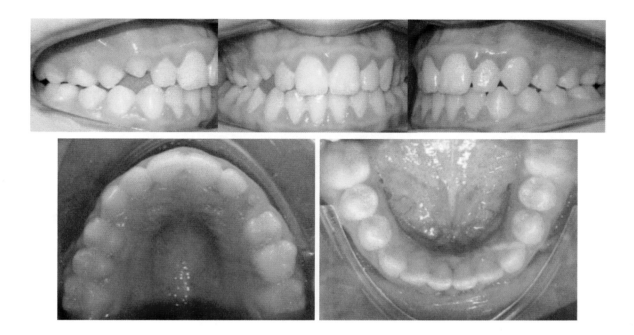

- Here we see how the shape of dental arches becomes broader and more rounded due to the modification of the position of the tongue; the patient is managing to correct breathing after the adenoid removal and the functional rehabilitation along with the Phonoaudiologist who collaborated in the treatment. The tongue itself in its correct position, removing the buccinator compressive action on the posterior alveolar ridges, and will contribute to the rehabilitation of the system.

BEFORE AND AFTER

As this is a growing patient, containment in this treatment will be the patient's own muscles, working properly. If the orthopedic treatment finished while the system is fully rehabilitated, there will be **NO** need for mechanical retainers.

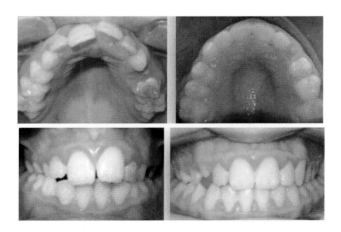

- Clinical case of an adolescent patient treated with Pitts 21. Class II is corrected with a mandibular advancement appliance (Twin Block) and the use of intermaxillary elastics; At the end of the treatment, the profile was improved due to the projection of the chin.

- As containment, it was decided to place a bimaxillary appliance (KEOA)

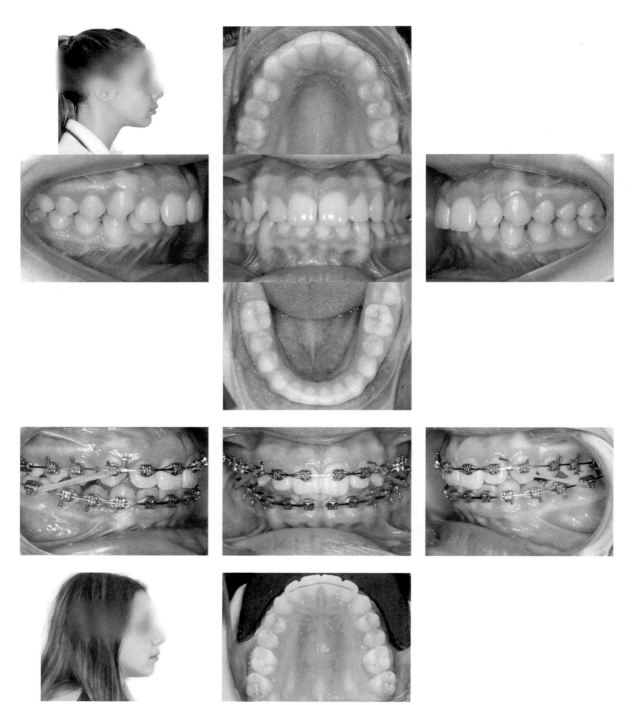

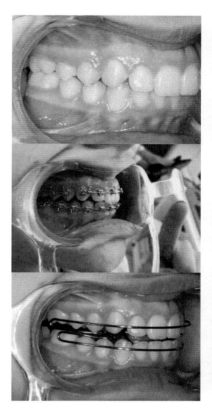
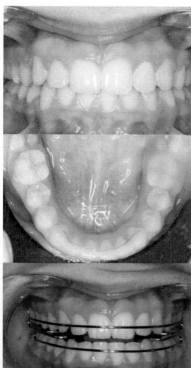
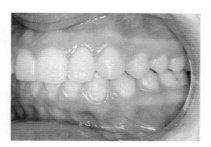
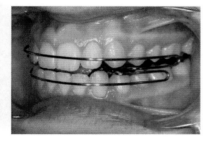

- This appliance as a containment should be used at night, and controlled by the professional over time to calibrate and place the buccal, palatal and acrylic arches correctly, avoiding any counterproductive effect caused by them when deformed inside the mouth during the daily use.

SWALLOWING

From birth to adulthood

Swallowing is the function developed after sucking or chewing. It involves facial, perioral, masticatory, supra and infrahyoid muscles.
There are 2 types of swallowing:

- Infant or primary swallowing

- Mature of secondary swallowing

INFANT OR PRIMARY SWALLOWING

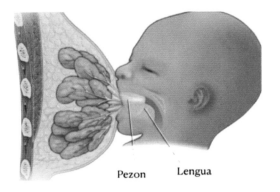

Pezon   Lengua

The baby uses the tongue as a reflex to express breast milk. The tongue advances between the lips with force to suck. The expanded tongue during the suction stimulates both, the development of the maxilla and the nasal breathing, since the infant will not be able to breathe through the mouth when it is occupied.

After 6 months will come the WEANING stage, where the ideal will be:

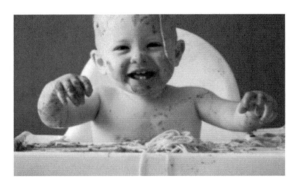

- "Real" food not processed, nor porridge
- Let them explore and choose
- Do not use teaspoon

When the stage of swallowing semi-solid and solid comes, concurrently with the appearance of the temporary teeth, there must be a CNS maturation in such a way that the pattern of primary or infant swallowing passes to the pattern of secondary or mature swallowing.

DEGLUCIÓN SECUNDARIA O MADURA

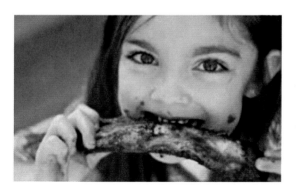

As the teeth appear, the swallowing pattern should evolve to a "MATURE" swallowing: the tongue pushes up against the palate, instead of going forward between the lips, which at this point would be between the teeth.

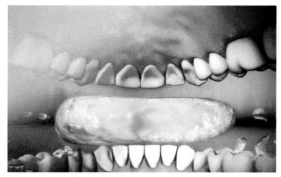

If primary swallowing persists while teeth are already in the mouth, then the balance will be disturbed and certain malocclusions will occur.

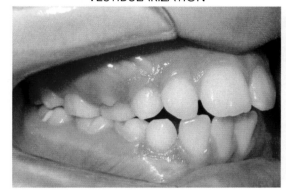

VESTIBULARIZATION

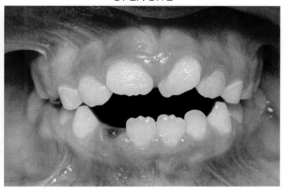

OPEN BITE

Clinical Case

8-year-old patient with atypical swallowing, lingual interposition between the dental arches which caused an anterior open bite.

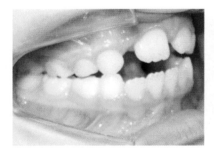
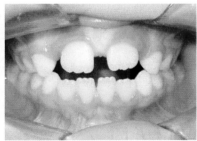
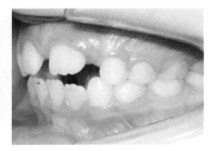

One of the therapeutic vehicles used for the functional rehabilitation of the tongue in atypical swallowing is the **BALTERS BIONATOR**, a rigid, bimaxillary device, which will have the purpose of relocating the tongue, so that the incisors can return to their position and establish the anterior guidance. It is a functional rehabilitator par excellence, for children of growing age and adults during containment following the orthodontic treatment, after the rehabilitation of open bite with a low friction with passive self- ligating philosophy (Pitts21).

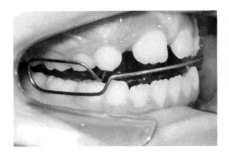 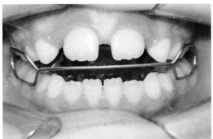 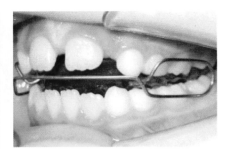

After 18 months the treatment is finished.

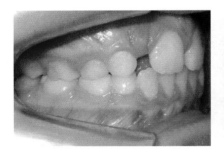 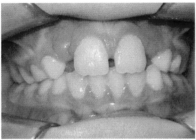 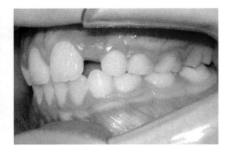

Pre and Post Treatment Images

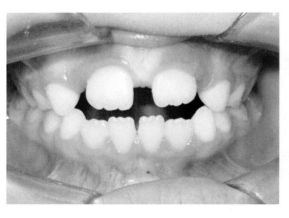 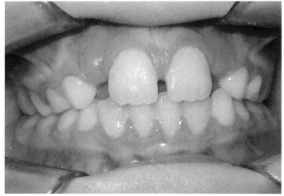

BALTERS BIONATOR

This device is composed of:

- Buccal arch

- Palatine arch or coffin

- Acrylic

Each part has a specific function that will rehabilitate each facial or masticatory muscle that is altered in its function

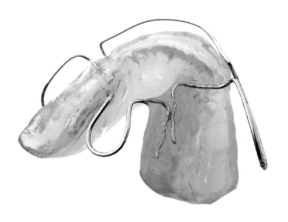

- **Buccal arch**:

  - In the anterior sector, it will be a rehabilitator of the bilabial closure, its function is that the patient manages to develop the necessary tonicity, trying to close with the upper and lower lip while touching this arch.

  - In the posterior sector, it will function as a "barrier" for the buccinator, which in these cases is in hypercontraction, cause narrow arches due to compression of the maxilla, as there is no balance between the external forces of this muscle and the internal forces represented by the tongue.

- **Palatine arch or coffin**: it is a rehabilitation of the lingual function, a reminder that lift the tongue to the palate to the correct place.

- **Acrylic:** in the anterior sector, it blocks the tongue from interposing in between the teeth preventing the persistence of the open bite and help incisors back to their position until they come into contact with each other (anterior guidance).

Clinical Case

Adult patient with open bite, treated with H4 low friction self-ligating bracket (Pitts21 brackets were not available yet), simultaneous biomechanics, ILSE, "squeezing exercises to tone the chewing muscles and perform posterior vertical control, and use of "lingual reminders" to rehabilitate the position of the tongue both at rest and in function.

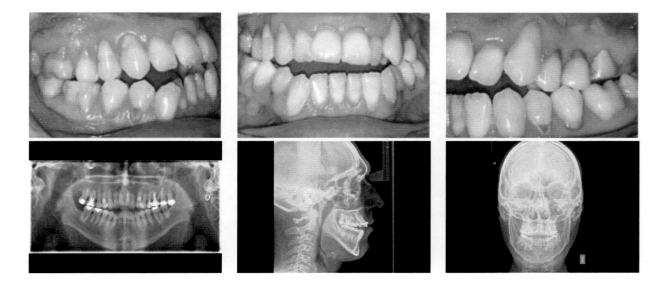

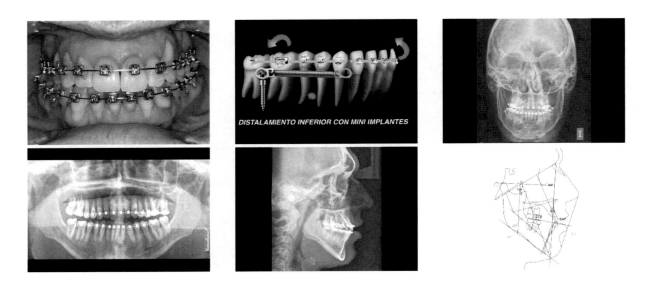

The patient is discharged after meeting all the objectives of the orthodontic treatment and it is suggested the use of a functional appliance as containment to "remind" the correct position and proper functioning to the perioral muscles, avoiding recurrences. The Balters Bionator was used every night to sleep and a few hours during the day.

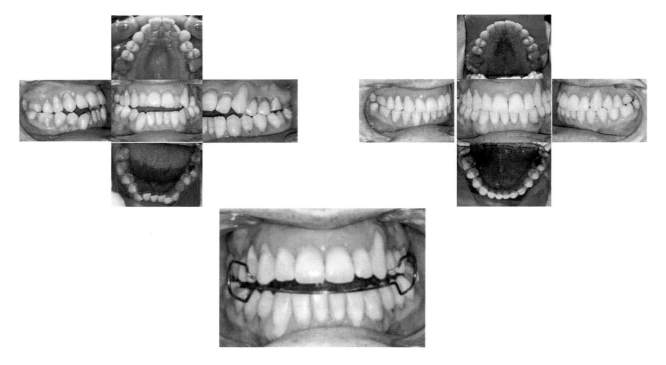

- The buccal arch in the anterior sector will function as a "LIP SEAL" training the lips to achieve closure without effort.

- The buccal arch in the posterior sector will separate the buccinators from the plastic zone of the dentoalveolar ridges.

- The acrylic will avoid the interposition of the tongue between the anterior teeth, "reminding" the tongue that this is not its place, but above where the "coffin" is.

Clinical Case

In this other case, an adult with atypical swallowing was treated with low friction self-ligating brackets with rectangular slot. During his mechanical treatment, we insisted on solving the functional part, since it was essential to remove the tongue that was interposed between the dental arches and generated the malocclusion.

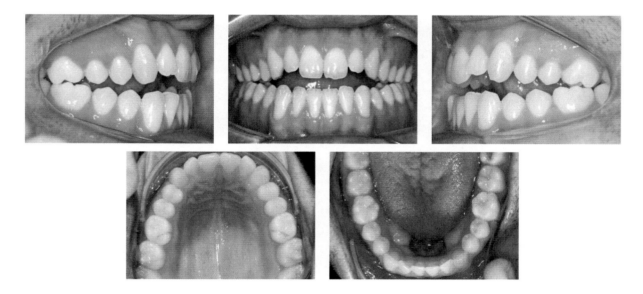

After 10 months of treatment, thanks to the advantages of low friction orthodontics with passive self-ligating in addition to the simultaneous biomechanics with broad archwires, disarticulations and "tongue lifting" exercises along with lingual reminders, and the use of ILSE (immediate light short elastics), the occlusal objective is achieved: return the lost anterior guidance, correct overjet and overbite and functional rehabilitation of the patient, eliminating one of the causal factors of the malocclusion.

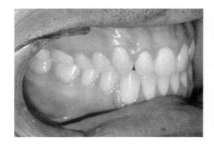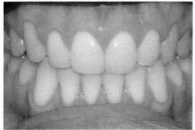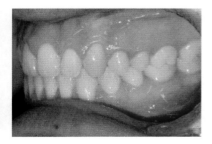

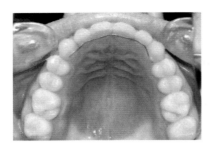
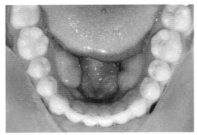

Once the appliances have been removed, regardless the fixed containment, we consider the importance of placing a vehicle that "reminds" the newly acquired tongue position, which will be essential as a factor for long-term stability. The patient is given a device from the Trainer system (T4 A), to be used at night when sleeping, and we recommend him to perform a series of exercises during the day.

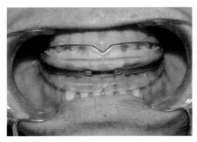
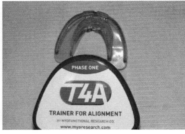
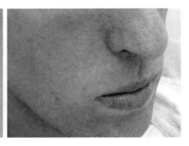

Clinical Case

A 13-year-old patient, with anterior open bite caused by lingual interposition during swallowing and low position at rest.
It is treated with low friction orthodontics, early elastics, broad archwires, and disarticulations with squeezing exercises.

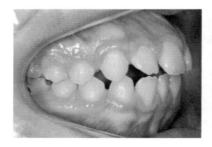
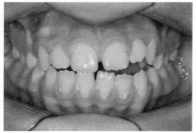
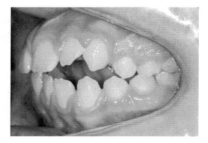

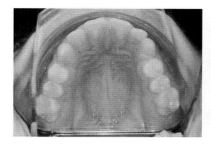 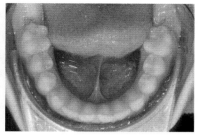

In the lateral teleradiography, we can see the tongue in a low position, evidenced by the straight line obtained when tracing the hyoid triangle.

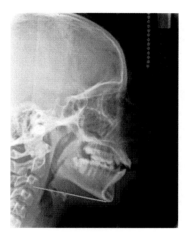

After removing the orthodontic appliances, regardless the fixed containment, we consider the importance of a bimaxillary containment device that helps to maintain or fully rehabilitates the swallowing function, and places the tongue in the correct position, preventing future recurrences.

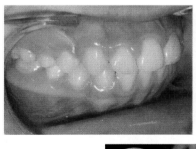 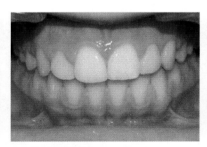 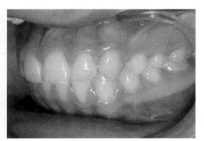

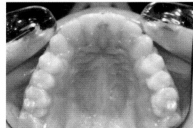 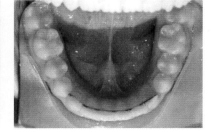

The chosen device was the BALTERS BIONATOR DE BALTERS for night use.

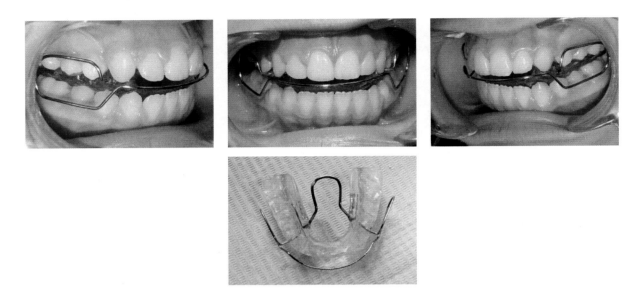

Clinical Case

A 10-year-old patient with a digital sucking habit, which causes a large anterior open bite and an atypical swallowing which enhances the dysfunction.

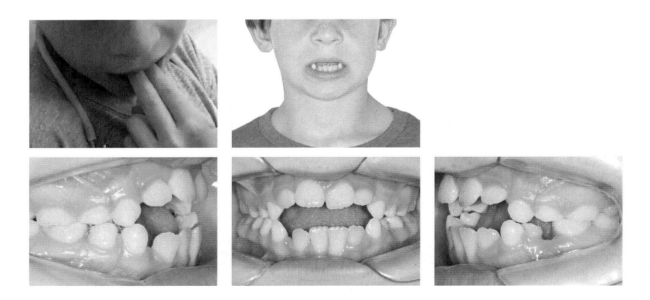

- We decided first to eliminate the habit of digital suction by placing a thumb crib, since it had to be resolved quickly and prior to orthodontics.

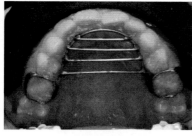

ORDER OF VEHICLES Ⓥ

- THUMB CRIB
- PITTS 21
- FUNCTIONAL DEVICE (KEOA.)

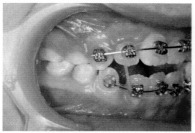 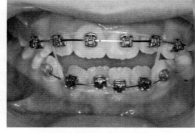 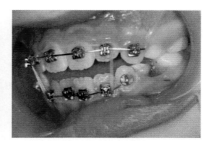

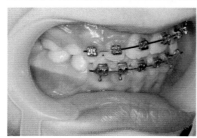 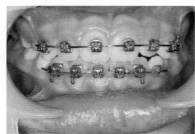 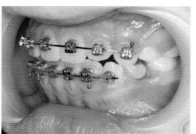

- After we finalized the phase 1 of the treatment, we achieved the closure of the anterior open bite and the anterior dental guidance was recovered; now we have the possibility of rehabilitating the swallowing.

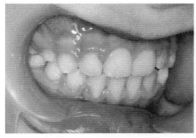 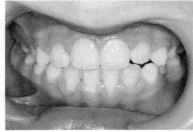 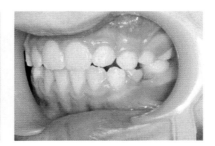

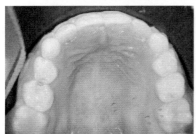 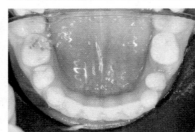

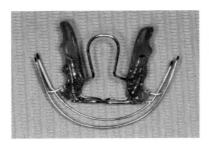 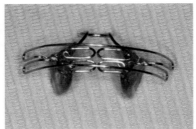 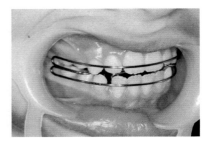

CHEWING

- Chewing is a function to consider as a possible factor of origin in certain early malocclusions and having repercussions in the adult.

- At 3 years of age, chewing matures with the passing from primary to secondary swallowing, where the masticatory muscles and the dentition participate.

- The onset or origin of some malocclusions in temporary dentition are in part directly related to the type of food the child eats. If this habit persists over time, the adults may have dentoalveolar and even facial consequences.

Heritage or Environment?

- And it is here that the question is posed: Will the dentoalveolar problems that we observe in the daily clinic at an early age, be of hereditary origin or will they be influenced by the environment?

- After reading extensive bibliographies, combined with many years of clinical experience, the answer makes me think that the development of the vast majority of problems draw influence from the environment, and if there were any predisposing genetic component present, undoubtedly the epigenetic factors will develop and enhance that condition.

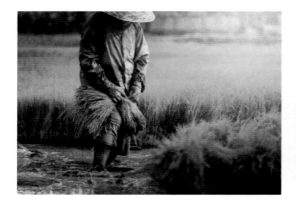 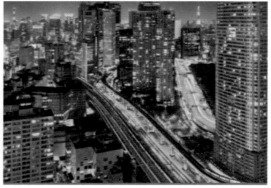

- There are studies that have genetically analyzed similar populations, living in contrasting environments, with different customs and eating habits. The general results showed that some of the orthodontic problems are of an environmental origin and not genetic. In rural environments, where the diet is based on **NON**-processed foods and little added sugar, it coincides with individuals with well-developed arches and low incidence of cavities; on the other hand, in large cities, individuals with small arches and a high cariogenic level are mostly observed.

RAW FOODS PROCESSED AND REFINED FOODS

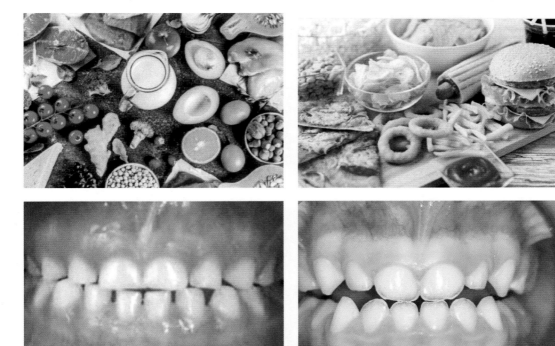

BROAD ARCH WITH DIASTEMAS   NARROW ARCH WITHOUT DIASTEMAS
(FUTURE CROWDING)

- In some cases, where the dental arches do not show physiological reductions resulting from a processed diet, the origin could possibly be **dental interference.**

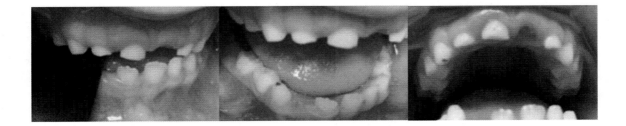

A dental interference that is not identified in time will generate the following malocclusions depending on the deviation in the final trajectory of mandibular closure:

- **Functional mandibular lateral deviation**: premature contact (usually canine), generates a displacement to the opposite side; it is clinically evidenced as a posterior unilateral crossbite.

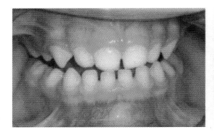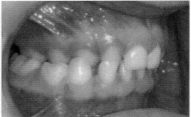

- **Functional anterior mandibular displacement**: premature contact generates a forward displacement of the mandible, shown as an anterior crossbite.

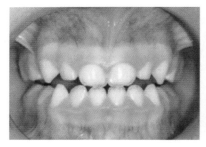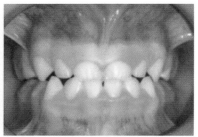

- But the story continues; not only does the soft or processed consistency of the food prevent the reduction of teeth generating dental interferences, but it also influences the development of the tonicity of the chewing muscles (mainly masseter and temporalis).

- It is also important to keep chewing in mind when diagnosing and treating adults orthodontically.

- It is very common to see a lack of masseter and temporalis muscle tonicity in patients who as children had a soft diet and did not develop their chewing muscles, and have brought the same habits into their adult life.

For this reason, in adults, during orthodontic treatment with Pitts21 passive self-ligating, ILSE and disarticulations, an indissoluble triad, it is extremely important to "train" these hypotonic muscles, allowing us to functionally rehabilitate the patient as their treatment advances.

Therapy Myofunctional in Treatment

- Myofunctional therapy consists of asking the patient to perform a series of exercises to increase the masseter and temporalis muscle tone, and thus achieve greater posterior vertical control.

- As Dr Pitts suggests in his care protocol and taking into account simultaneous biomechanics, these exercises shall be performed by the patient at the beginning of their orthodontic treatment.

MYOFUNCTIONAL THERAPY

- Masseter
- Temporalis

SQUEEZING EXERCISES

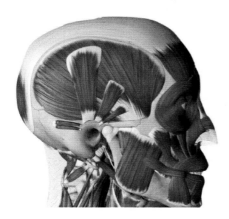 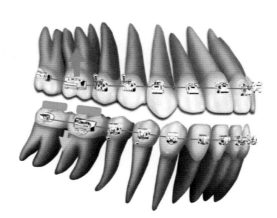

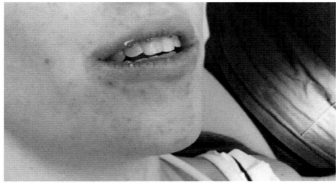

- The "Squeezing" exercises consist of: squeezing the disarticulations that we place in the molar area for 60 uninterrupted seconds tightly, 6 times a day, taking note of how the masseter and temporary contraction are marked on the face.

- Another type of tightening consists of the "6 x 6 x 6" technique, which is to squeeze the molar area 6 times, for 6 seconds, 6 times a day.

APPENDIX OF RECOMMENDED EXERCISES FOR MYOFUNCTIONAL THERAPY

The Foggy Mirror

The patient is instructed to inhale air through both nostrils deeply and place a mirror under the nose. Then when he exhales, he should see if the mirror has fogged up. Inhale air again, now through a single nostril and place the mirror again under that nostril to see if it has fogged up; Repeat this action with the other nostril individually.

Stimulating Tubes

The patient is instructed to place a stimulator tube in each nostril and with the lips completely closed, he should breathe only through these tubes.

Conscious Breathing

In this therapy, the patient is instructed to do the following exercise so that he learns to identify the type of breathing he has; if it is superficial or deeper at the lung level (ideal).

The patient will learn to breathe only through the nose, without moving the shoulders, or the chest only by moving the abdomen.

He should practice it using 3 different postures:

- Sitting: sitting on a bench that does not have a back, with his posture being of an upright nature and his feet touching the floor. He should inhale and exhale slowly only moving his abdomen.

- Sticking to the wall: with the right posture, the patient should stick his back towards the wall, exaggerate his posture and also stick his shoulders to the wall. Once this posture is adopted, he should inhale slowly and exhale only with movement of the abdomen.

- Lying on the floor: when lying on the floor, the patient should rest his shoulders on the floor, place an object (box, ball, book) on his abdomen and see how it rises when breathing only with the movement of the abdomen, without there being movement of the shoulders or of the chest.

LIP THERAPIES

Blowing up the Balloon

Here we must instruct the patient to take a latex balloon and inflate it by blowing into it without touching it with their hands; the balloon shall be held by the lips only.

Lip Pops

In this exercise we ask the patient to take in air through their mouth, seal their lips, and inflate their cheeks to release the air in the form of a Pop or bubble (the "Pop" sound should be heard).

Blowfish

We ask the patient to take in air through their mouth and inflate the cheeks and lips, pushing the air out while keeping the lips sealed to prevent the air from escaping. The patient should feel the air pressure on your muscles.

Buttons

In this technique, the patient is asked to place the largest button inside the mouth between the teeth and the lips, then they must close their lips, push the button out horizontally, down and up while trying to keep it inside their mouth. Then they repeat the same exercise with the medium button and finally with the smallest button.

Holding Straws or Cookies

The patient is asked to place a straw or cookie between the lips and should keep it horizontal for 1 minute, preventing it from moving, and always try to keep it horizontal.

Moving the Lips

Make a movement with your lips to the right side and to the left side, reaching the farthest position you can on each side.

Holding the Spoon

The patient is asked to hold a spoon with his lips and keep it horizontal without moving it, then he can place weight on the spoon (coins or some object) and he will try to keep it horizontal, holding it with his lips only.

Suck and Hold

The patient is asked to stick the tip of the tongue in the resting position and then the entire tongue on the roof of the mouth (palate), suck and hold the tongue against the roof of the mouth for 1 minute.

Moving the Tongue

We ask the patient to stick their tongue out as far forward as possible, then move the tongue to the right side without touching the edge of the mouth (corner of the mouth) and finally move it to the left side.

Sweeping the Palate

To perform this technique, you need to have a hand mirror. You are asked to stick the tip of the tongue in the resting position and then to sweep the roof of the mouth (palate) with the tip of the tongue, from front to back, repeat constantly.

Counter resistance

The patient is asked to stick the tongue out and force it outward, while a tongue depressor applies resistance to the tip of the tongue; you should feel pressure on your tongue muscles.

Pushing the Palate

With a piece of chewing gum on the tip of the tongue, we ask the patient to stick and push the tip of the tongue in the resting position; then we ask him to lift the tip of his tongue and force it upwards, pressing the gum against the palatal ridges.

Tip of the Tongue Up

The patient is asked to fully stick the tongue out and lift the tip upward without touching either of the lips.

THERAPIES FOR THE PROPER SWALLOWING:

Swallow Without Moving the Lips

We ask the patient to swallow several times while standing in front of the mirror, and to not make any movement with the lower lip while swallowing.

Funny Face Swallow

Here we will ask the patient to swallow by relaxing the muscles and refrain from movement on their face or lips.

Swallow with Spray (squirt bottle swallow)

This exercise can be done with the patient in the office chair. We ask him to place his tongue in the resting position, spray the floor of his mouth, and then ask him to swallow without removing the tip of his tongue from the resting position.

Reflex Swallowing

The patient should hold the tip of the tongue and at the same time, cold water will be injected into the palate with a syringe. This will be swallowed with the back of the palate and the veil producing the A phoneme.

Reflex Swallowing

We ask the patient to put the tip of the tongue in a resting position, take a sip of water and put the tongue in the shape of a spoon to hold the water in the center, close with his posterior teeth and start swallowing properly, while keeping his head elevated, and then tilt his head back to swallow the last drop. The patient should not lick his lips after he drinks.

CHEWING THERAPIES:

Over Chewing

We ask the patient to chew each bite of the food on both sides of his mouth 15 times, keeping count in his mind.

Chewing Gum

We ask the patient to chew the gum on both sides of their mouth for 2 minutes.

SECTION 3

ASYMMETRIES AND ASYMMETRIC BIOMECHANICS

Section 3
Asymmetries and Asymmetric Biomechanics
Chapter 8
Introduction

Before distances were greater because space is measured by time
Jorge Luis Borges (1899-1986)
Argentine writer and poet.

The cases of asymmetries provide us with variants in their Diagnosis **D** and, consequently, the Planning/Vehicles **P.V**, and Biomechanics **B** for their treatment also differ from each other.

We can schematically classify them into dental, functional, skeletal, and another group that combines, in the same case, 2 and even 3 of the above-mentioned variants.

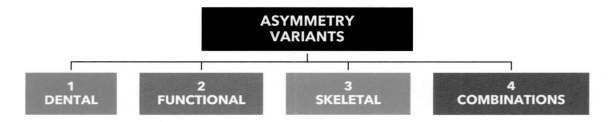

1

1) DENTAL ASYMMETRIES

The dental asymmetries correspond to tooth-bone discrepancy problems; they can appear at any age, that is, in "early" treatments of Phase I of mixed dentition, or Phase II of teenagers and adults. Generally, they have a favorable prognosis as long as the missing spaces, the spaces to be maintained, or the spaces to be closed are properly treated.

Figures 2 to 11 show images of 2 dental asymmetries, one of them with lack of space for tooth # 12; the other, with anterior diastemas derived from the agenesis of the upper right lateral incisor; both patients present, though with different causes and treatments, dental asymmetries with maxillary right midline deviation.

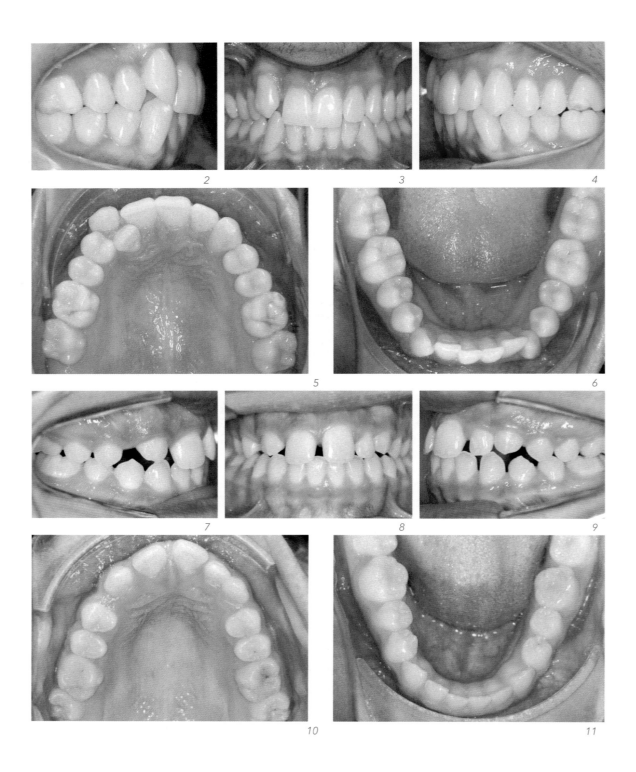

2 *3* *4*

5 *6*

7 *8* *9*

10 *11*

The causes of these frequent problems can be from different primary etiologies that, over time, lead us to dental asymmetries. *(Fig. 12)*

DENTAL ASYMMETRIES / ETIOLOGIES
A. INSUFFICIENT SPACE FOR CORRECT DENTAL POSITIONING
B. ECTOPIC ERUPTIONS
C. SUPERNUMERARIES
D. AGENESIS
E. CYSTS
F. ANKYLOSES
G. RETAINED TEETH
H. INTERPROXIMAL CAVITIES
I. LOSS OF TEETH
J. DIFFERENCE IN M-D SIZE IN CONTRALATERAL TEETH

12

2) FUNCTIONAL ASYMMETRIES

In early treatments (Phase I), as well as in teenagers or adults (Phase II), a group of patients in maximum intercuspation will present an orthopedic imbalance in their TMJ with mandibular functional displacement.

At first, it is possible that the mandibular closure, guided by muscles, ligaments and other articular components, can be seen as being hampered by a certain occlusal interference that, when "avoided", generates, in time and under repetition, a neuromuscular response with maximum intercuspation of greater comfort at the expense of an orthopedic instability of the TMJ. *(Figs. 13 and 14)*

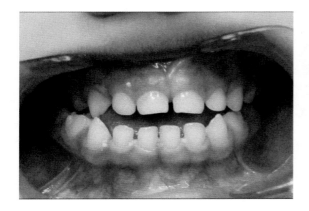 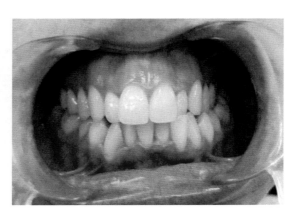

13   14

FUNCTIONAL ASYMMETRIES
MANDIBULAR DEFLECTION
ETIOLOGY

A. **DENTAL MALPOSITION THAT GENERATES DEFLECTIVE CONTACT**

B. **TRANSVERSE ARCH DISCREPANCY**

C. **INADEQUATE INCLINATION (TORQUE) IN THE PREMOLAR(S) AND/OR MOLAR(S) SECTOR**

3) SKELETAL ASYMMETRIES

Another group of patients, apart from their malocclusion, present a varied backdrop for their asymmetry that we have to assess in the diagnosis, prognosis, treatment plan and execution; in them, we find different shapes and condyle sizes, vertical offsets in maxilla, canted plane occlusal, etc., etc.

In these cases, after a general diagnosis **D**, it is crucial to know what kind of expectations the patients have for their treatment; do they want to improve their dental aesthetic and occlusion? (camouflage solution) or, do they wish for a macro aesthetic change?

In this chapter we will discuss two patients of female sex, similar age, with skeletal asymmetries, who opted for different options.

3.A) Camouflage option *(Figs. 15 to 54)*

3.B) Orthodontics + orthognathic surgery option *(Figs. 59 and 86)*

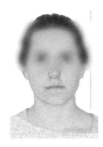

15   16   17

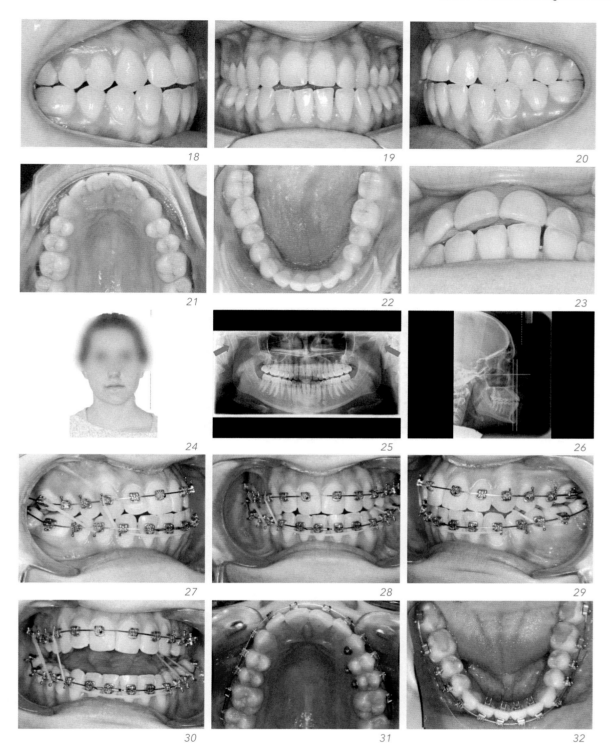

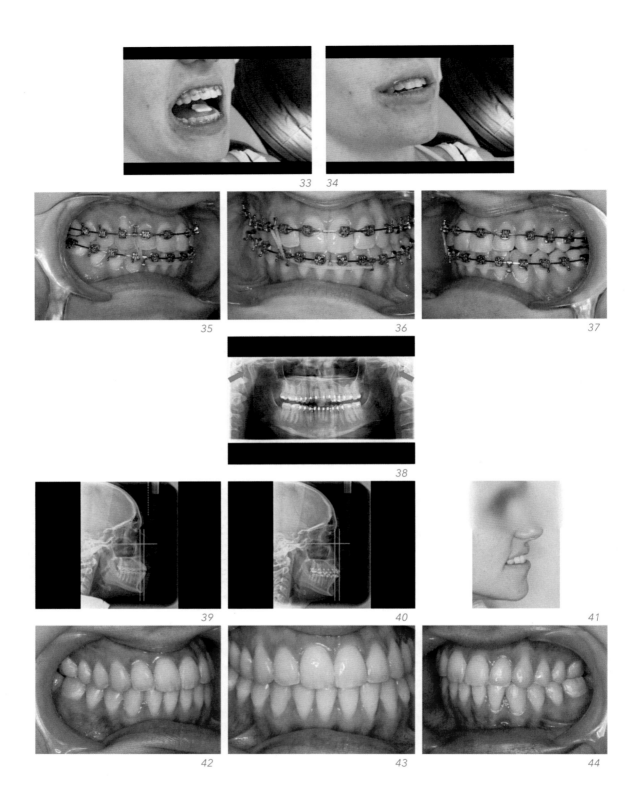

33 34

35 36 37

38

39 40 41

42 43 44

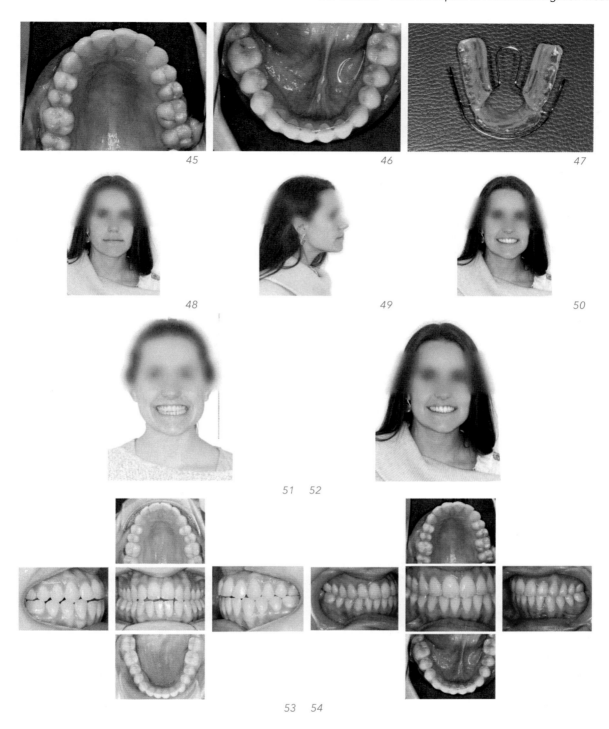

45   46   47

48   49   50

51   52

53   54

3.A) Camouflage option (Figs. 15 to 54)

D This patient, in addition to her open bite, presented a clinically appreciable skeletal asymmetry. The panoramic X-ray confirmed it (see mandibular condyles). Her treatment requirements were related to SAP correction since she has a reverse curve of smile and occlusal functionalities.

P.V A «camouflage» treatment was planned with PSL Pitts 21 with "Flipped" brackets (180° turn) in upper incisors and Simultaneous Asymmetric Biomechanics.

B An archwire progression of .018 x .018 and .020 x .020 NiTi Ultra Soft Pitts Broad followed by.020 x .020 B Titanium with posts; the placement of elastics was always asymmetrical.

SKELETAL ASYMMETRIES MORE COMMON ETIOLOGIES
A. **GENETIC OR CONGENITAL**
B. **MANDIBLE MACRO-TRAUMA IN GROWING PATIENTS**
C. **FUNCTIONAL DEVIATIONS IN GROWTH STAGE**
D. **ACQUIRED FACTORS.** **Examples: INFECTIONS, TUMORS, DEGENERATIVE PROCESSES AT THE CONDYLES, ETC.**

3.B) Orthodontics + orthognathic surgery option

SKELETAL	+	DENTAL

(Figs. 55 y 84)

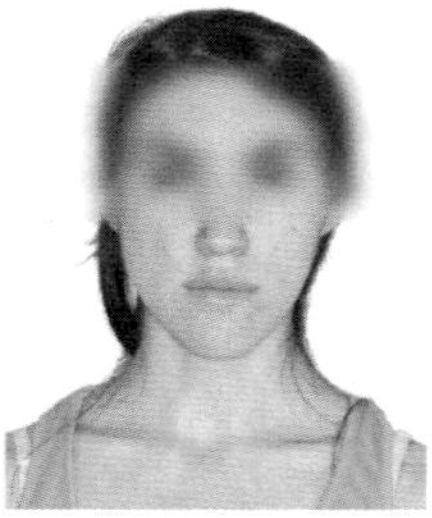

55

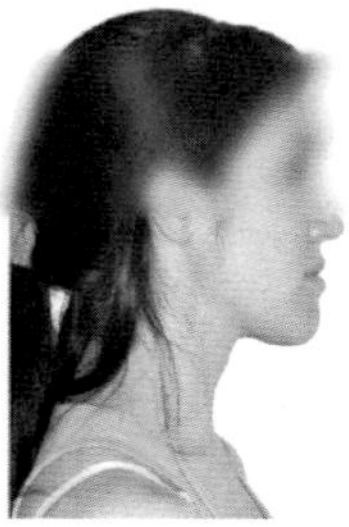

56

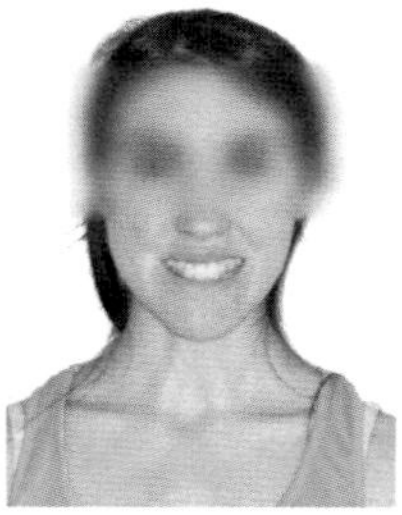

57

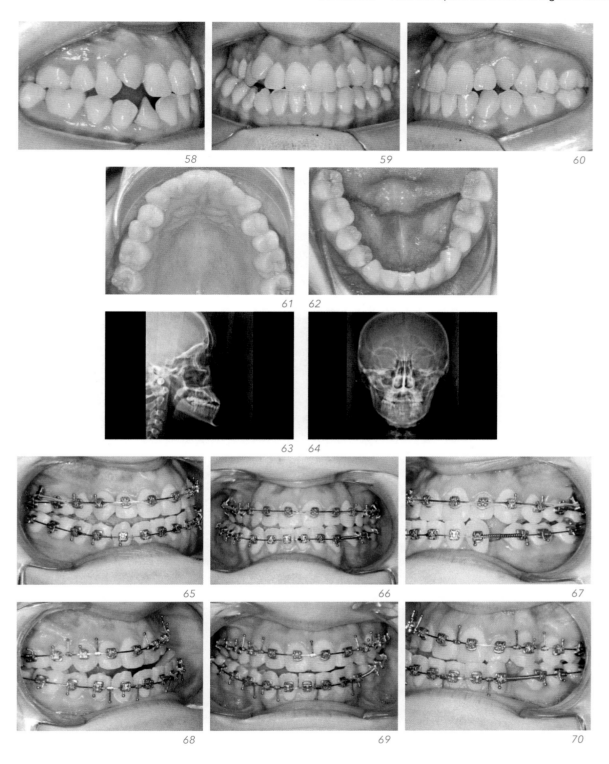

58   59   60

61   62

63   64

65   66   67

68   69   70

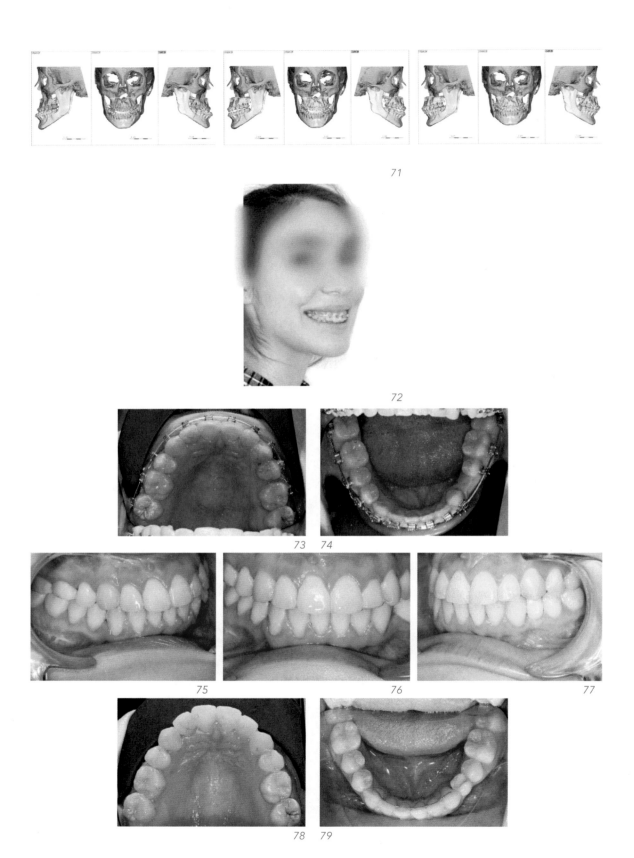

71

72

73   74

75   76   77

78   79

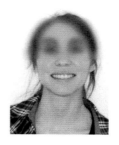
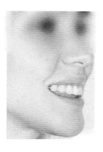
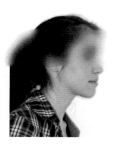

80 *81* *82*

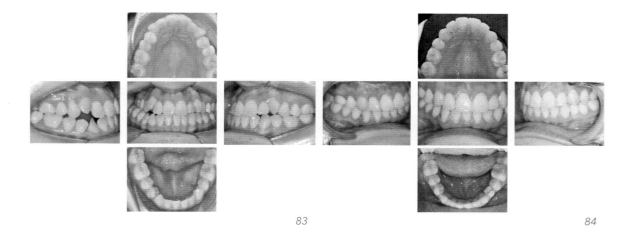

83 *84*

This young patient presented a skeletal asymmetry that, orthodontically, they had wanted to resolve with the extraction of tooth 34 (1st left lower premolar), thus generating a dental asymmetry.

Her requirements before the treatment were to improve the aesthetic aspects of her smile, but also macro aesthetics improvements.

Considering the diagnosis, , we chose an orthodontic-surgical-implant treatment plan **P** that would include the extraction of upper second premolars and an anterosuperior retraction with maximum anchorage.

In the lower arch, we opened space for an implant of the tooth # 34 that had been extracted.
These procedures would be complemented with a surgery that would involve both the maxilla and the mandible.

In Biomechanics **B**, presurgical orthodontics were performed using tubes and H4 brackets (PSL), also the anterosuperior retraction using infrazygomatic TADS and elastic chain. *(Figs. 55 and 84)*
The orthognathic surgery and the implant were performed by Dr. Claudio Fernández (Uruguay).

4) COMBINATIONS

We have already pointed out that the other asymmetries that we see at our office combine 2 and, on occasions, 3 of the mentioned variants.

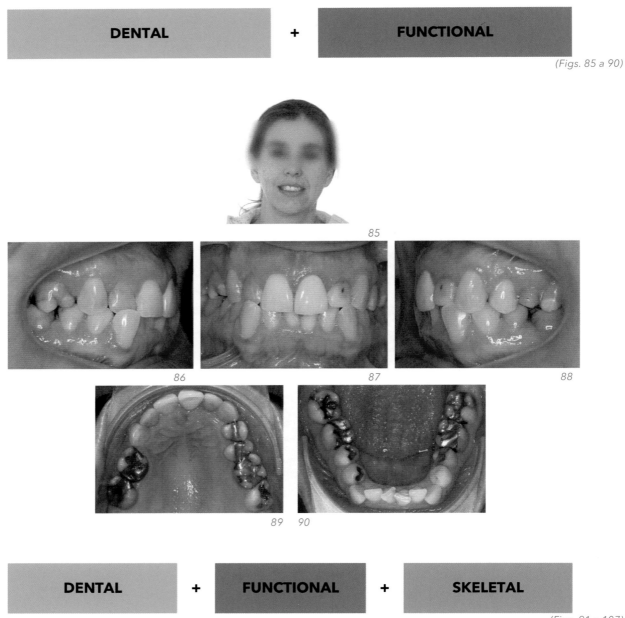

DENTAL + **FUNCTIONAL**

(Figs. 85 a 90)

85

86   87   88

89   90

DENTAL + **FUNCTIONAL** + **SKELETAL**

(Figs. 91 a 107)

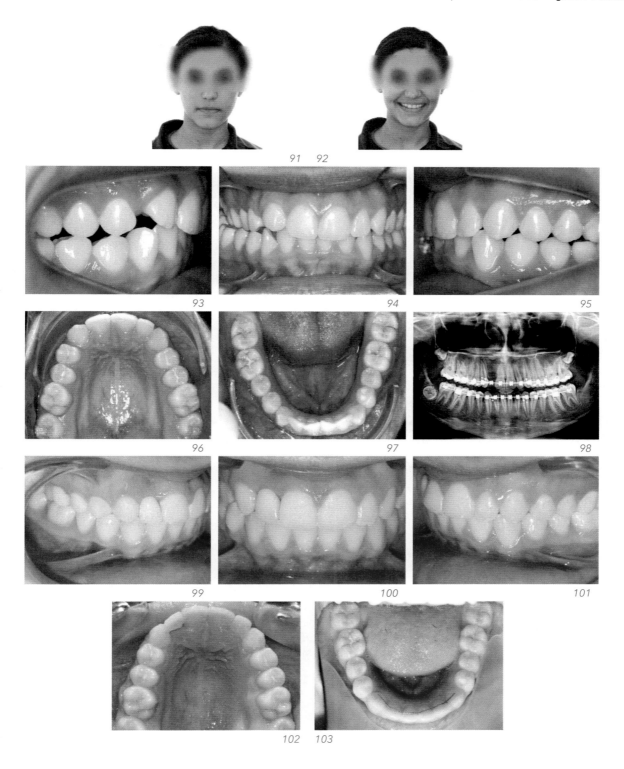

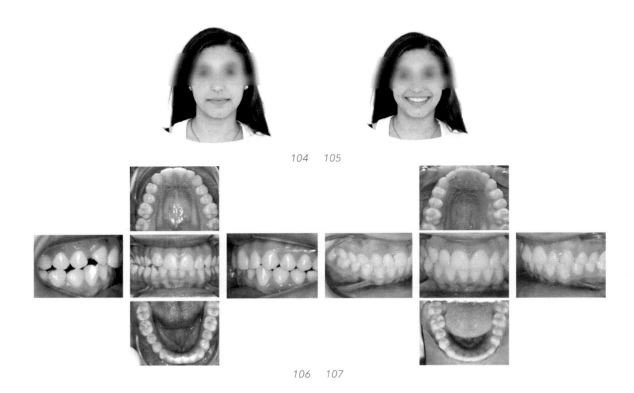

104   105

106   107

B

SIMULTANEOUS BIOMECHANICS

When we approach, plan and execute treatments of different asymmetries, typically the Biomechanical **B** responses are also asymmetric. *(Figs 108 and 109)*

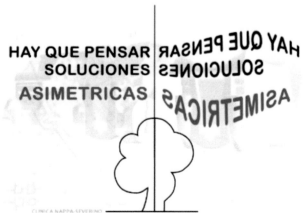

HAY QUE PENSAR
SOLUCIONES
ASIMETRICAS

108

VARIANTS

A. LINKS

B. SPRINGS

C. ELASTICS

D. EXTRACTIONS

E. INTERPROXIMAL REDUCTIONS - I.P.R.

F. IMPLANTS

G. T.A.D.S.

H. SURGERY

109

We are going to see some of these variants in the cases presented in this section.

Section 3

Asymmetries and Asymmetric Biomechanics

Chapter 9

Patient 5

Somewhere, something incredible is waiting to be known.
Carl Sagan (1934-1996)
American astronomer and writer.

As we established in the introduction to the section (Chapter 8), from the diagnostic point of view (D), there are dental, functional and skeletal asymmetries, while some present a combination of 2 or even 3 of these variants.

The case that we present here combines a small skeletal asymmetry with a more notable functional asymmetry. *(Figs 1 and 15)*

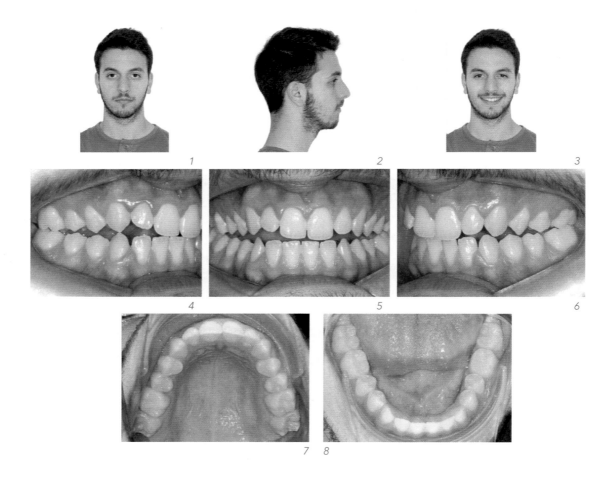

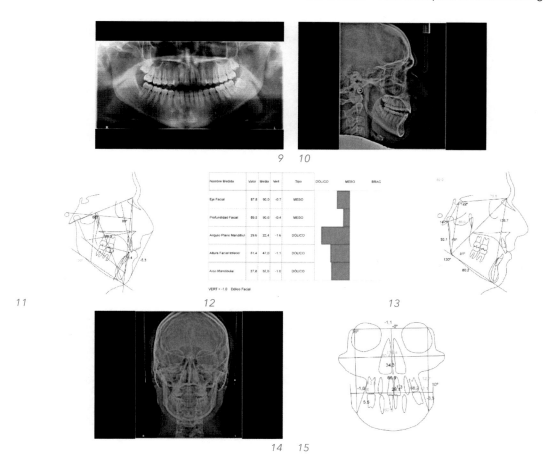

9 10

11   12   13

14 15

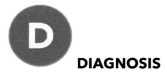

DIAGNOSIS

Checking areas that we have already mentioned, we were collecting, in an orderly manner, the profile of our patient's orthodontic problems. *(Figs 16)*

1) AGE AND BIOTYPE

2) AESTHETIC

3) SKELETAL

4) DENTAL

5) FUNCTIONAL

6) PATIENT REQUIREMENTS

16

1) AGE AND BIOTYPE

A young adult, and so, the incidence in favor or against growth was not a factor to consider.

2) AESTHETIC

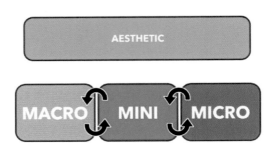

17

In macro, vertically, the lower third of the face exceeds the middle. **(RED)**

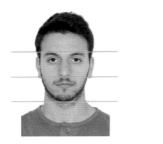 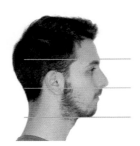

18   19

Increased nasolabial angle and short neck-chin distance.
The smile shows a reverse curve with canines much longer than lateral incisors. SAP **(blue)** *(Fig. 20)*

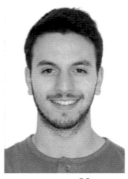

20

3) SKELETAL

There was a small asymmetry that was combined with a mandibular functional deviation in maximum intercuspation. *(Figs. 1, 11 and 15)*

4) DENTARY

In maximum intercuspation (MI), there were few interarch contact points with open bite in lateral sectors and insufficient anterior guidance found.

Very poor maximum intercuspation that shows us in the frontal view a misalignment of upper and lower midline, as well as the typical "hourglass" with dentoalveolar narrowing due to muscle imbalances. *(Figs. 21 a 25)*

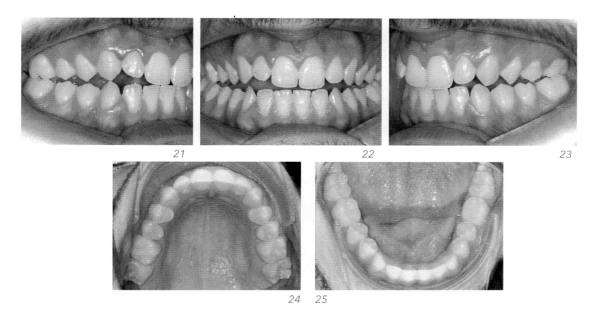

21   22   23

24   25

The panoramic X-ray shows the absence of tooth # 48 (it had been extracted), while tooth # 38 was semi-retained and badly positioned due to lack of space; the upper third molars also showed certain eruptive problems; this issue continued in the post-treatment and the extractions of these 3 teeth were recommended. *(Figs. 26 y 27)*

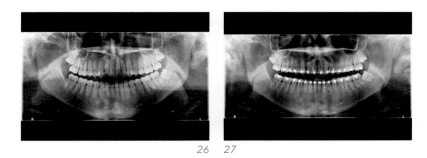

26   27

5) FUNCTIONAL

Due to occlusal interferences, a mandibular deviation to right was noticeable in maximum intercuspation.

Photographs 28 and 29 show the midline misalignments between both arches in maximum intercuspation *(Fig. 28)* that was reduced with a certain mouth opening and eliminating the deflective contacts. *(Fig. 29)*

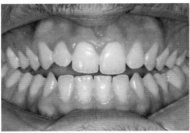 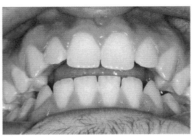

28 29

Joining concepts of the dental and functional areas, we noticed an orthopedic imbalance of the TMJ caused by a very bad inter-arch occlusal relationship. The lateral X-ray shows a vertical positioning of the hyoid at the level of the lower edge of the 4th vertebra, which is consistent with possible contractures of the infra hyoid muscles, a low lingual positioning and its lateral interposition in swallowing. *(Fig. 30)*

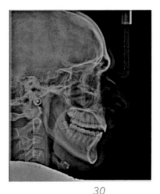

30

6) PATIENT REQUIREMENTS

The patient was referred to our clinic by a colleague who checked him during a routine check-up and warned him of his occlusal-functional problems.

He did not like his smile much, and the reserve curve was evident, that is a highly insufficient arc. SAP **(blue)** *(Fig. 31)*

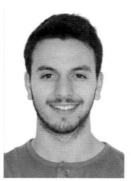

31

Since we made the (D) diagnosis, it was clear that we should plan a treatment essentially for a functional asymmetry case but also with a small skeletal incidence.

PLANNING AND THERAPEUTIC VEHICLES (PV)

The necessary corrections to be made referring to the aesthetic, transversal, vertical and, fundamentally, the combined asymmetries required simultaneous biomechanics that would be fulfilled with the triple vehicular association (V) of:

1. **PITTS 21 (FOR ITS EARLY AND EFFECTIVE 3D CONTROL)**

2. **IMMEDIATE ASYMMETRIC ELASTICS (ILSE)**

3. **DISARTICULATIONS**

We want to record that in this case the disarticulations were essential to:

A. **MUSCLE DEPROGRAMMING**

B. **PROMOTE THE DEVELOPMENT OF THE ARCHES**

C. **ENHANCE THE ASYMMETRIC EFFECT OF THE ELASTICS TO BE USED**

(Figs. 32 a 38)

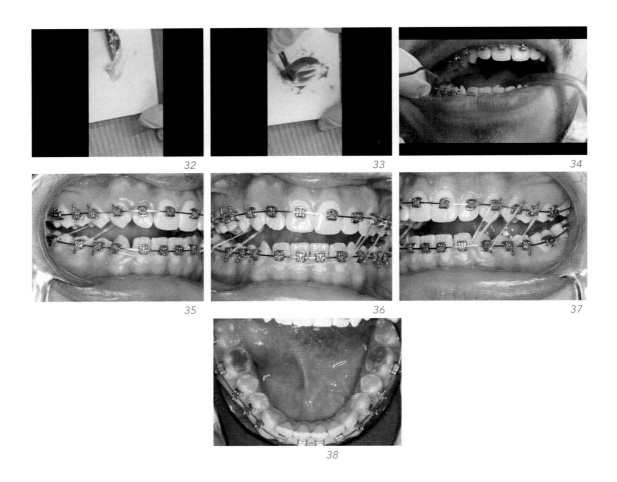

32 *33* *34*

35 *36* *37*

38

B SIMULTANEOUS BIOMECHANICS

1. **PITTS 21**
2. **MUSCLE DEPROGRAMMING**
3. **DEVELOPMENT OF THE ARCHES**
4. **IMMEDIATE ASYMMETRIC ELASTICS (ILSE)**
5. **NEUROMUSCULAR EXERCISES**

1) PITTS 21

Due to a slight retro inclination of teeth # 11 and 21 as well as a proclination of teeth # 12 and 22, the standard torque was used in all the teeth except for the latter 2, which were rotated 180°. *(Figs. 39 a 53)*

Once again, we emphasize the -27° of the upper molar tubes, and their importance in the interarch transverse coordination.

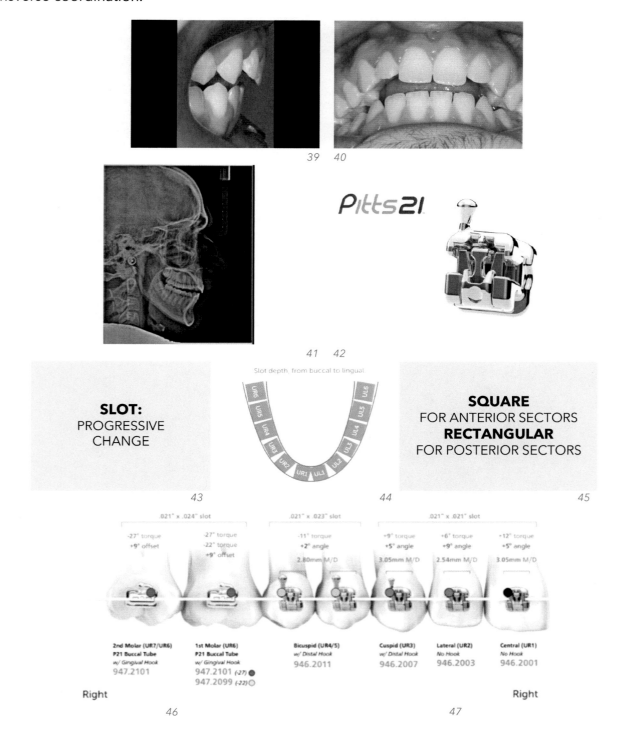

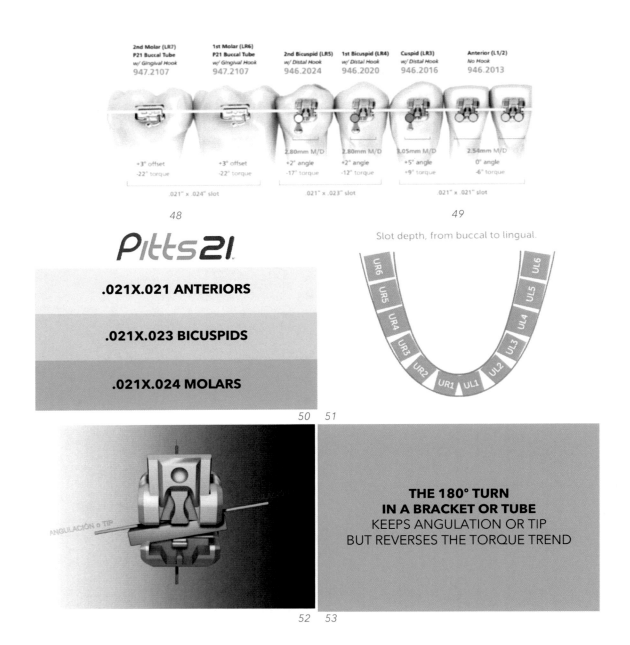

| 2nd Molar (LR7) P21 Buccal Tube w/ Gingival Hook 947.2107 | 1st Molar (LR6) P21 Buccal Tube w/ Gingival Hook 947.2107 | 2nd Bicuspid (LR5) w/ Distal Hook 946.2024 | 1st Bicuspid (LR4) w/ Distal Hook 946.2020 | Cuspid (LR3) w/ Distal Hook 946.2016 | Anterior (L1/2) No Hook 946.2013 |

| +3° offset -22° torque | +3° offset -22° torque | 2.80mm M/D +2° angle -17° torque | 2.80mm M/D +2° angle -12° torque | 3.05mm M/D +5° angle +9° torque | 2.54mm M/D 0° angle -6° torque |

.021" x .024" slot   .021" x .023" slot   .021" x .021" slot

48   49

Pitts21

.021X.021 ANTERIORS

.021X.023 BICUSPIDS

.021X.024 MOLARS

Slot depth, from buccal to lingual.

50   51

ANGULACIÓN o TIP

THE 180° TURN IN A BRACKET OR TUBE KEEPS ANGULATION OR TIP BUT REVERSES THE TORQUE TREND

52   53

2) NEUROMUSCULAR DEPROGRAMMING

The information from interfering occlusal contacts "travels" to the central nervous system, and the neuromuscular response tends to avoid them by laterally deflecting the mandible in this case to right. *(Fig. 54)*

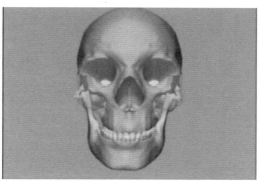

54

As it was established in (PV), this is a first objective of the disarticulations in functional asymmetries, "erasing" that information that also varies during treatment due to the positional changes of teeth with the progression of archwires.

3) DEVELOPMENT OF ARCH

4) IMMEDIATE ASYMMETRIC ELASTICS (ILSE)

We have joined these 2 sections but along with the Pitts 21 (PSL) and the disarticulations, they form a set in which they all enhance and reinforce each other.

After 3 weeks with upper and lower NiTi .014 Pitts Broad archwires, we switched both arches to .018 x .018 NiTi Ultra Soft Pitts Broad; a key factor in this case, for both the transverse and anteroposterior development of the arches, and the enormous progress in 3D control of the teeth.

The side elastics were different in arrangement but equal in diameter and force (3/16" and 2.5 oz); on the right side, they were used from lingual buttons on premolars to hooks on # 45 and 46, that is, through the arch, enhancing the transversal dentoalveolar effect in the upper right quadrant.

On the left side, with the same diameter and force (3/16" and 2.5 oz), elastics were inserted into upper premolars while in the lower left arch were in canine and first premolar.

In the anterior sector, the use of a 5/16" elastic, 2 ½ oz in reverse L was indicated in teeth # 43 - 32 and 23.

These Simultaneous and asymmetric Biomechanics are shown between *photographs 55 a 65*.

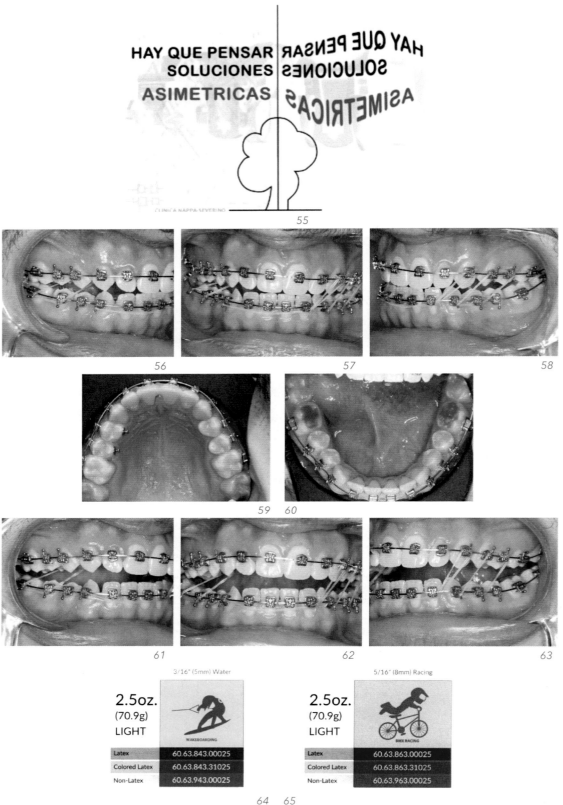

ASIMETRICAS

~ 182 ~

After 3 months of treatment, archwires progressed to.020 x .020 NiTi Pitts Broad; the elastics changed to be 3/16" but with 3.5 oz used per buccal surface in all 4 quadrants. *(Figs. 66 to 71)*

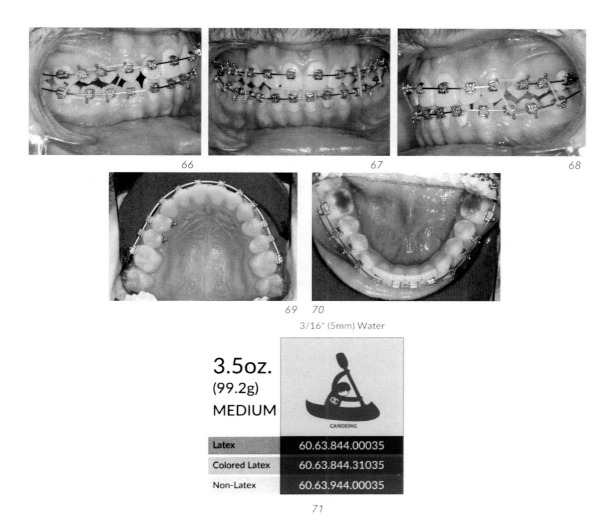

3/16" (5mm) Water

71

We followed with .20 x .020 B titanium archwires with «crimped» posts between lateral incisors and canines.

The elastics, asymmetrical in their disposition, were short Class II in the right sector and short Class III in the left sector; both 3/16" diameter and 3.5 oz (99 grs.) of force. *(Figs. 72 to 79)*

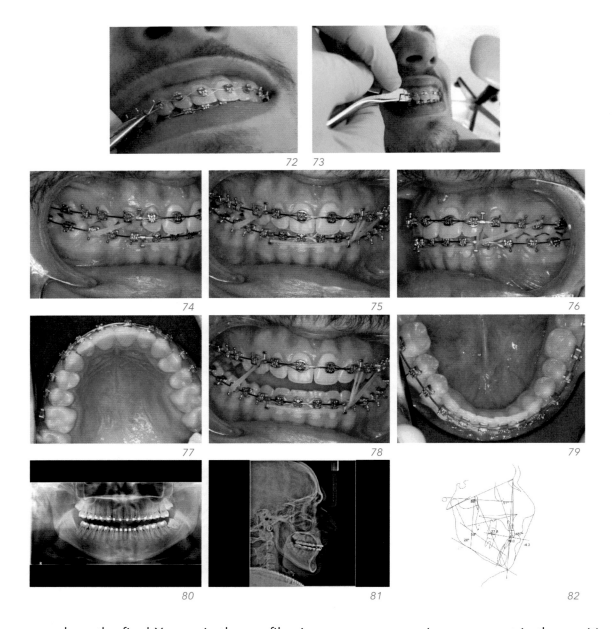

Figures. 80 to 82 show the final X-rays; in the profile view we can see an improvement in the positioning of the hyoid and a good upper incisor inclination.

Fig. 83 to 91 show dental and facial photographs at the end of the active treatment.

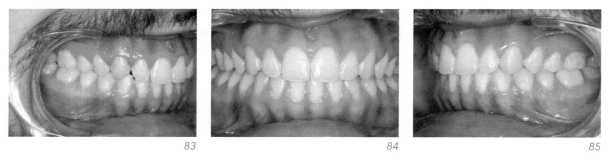

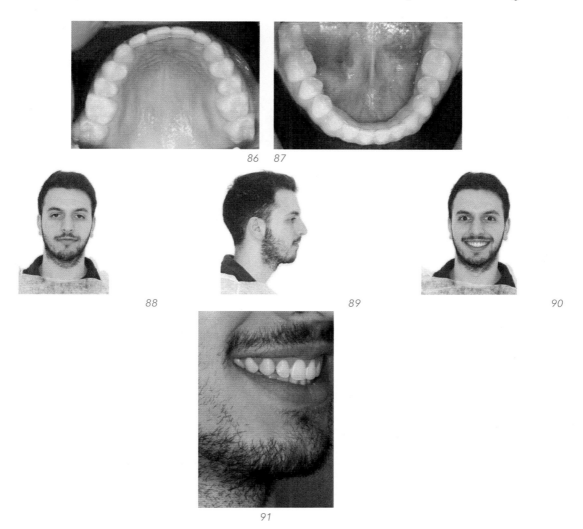

86 87

88   89   90

91

The small incisor reduction of his upper canines improved and allowed the design of a correct smile arch (SAP), but did not affect the functional objective of these teeth to be a guide of disocclusion of mandibular lateral movements. *(Figs. 92 to 93)*

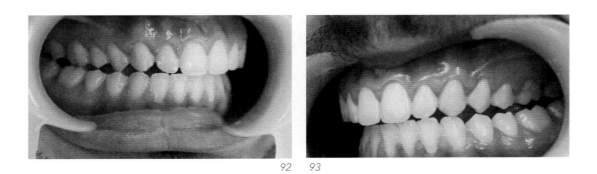

92   93

Section 3
Asymmetries and Asymmetric Biomechanics
Chapter 10
Patient 6

"I Hear and I Forget, I See and I Remember, I Do and I Understand"
Confucius (551-479 A.C.)
Chinese thinker.

This case is a singular and very small double asymmetry, on the one hand, a dental asymmetry with an upper midline slightly deviated to left and, on the other hand, a functional asymmetry with a mandibular deflection to right as a result of interfering occlusal contacts.

This case, actually, deserves to be in the aesthetic section (Section 1) since the great and special requirements of the patient belonged to that area.

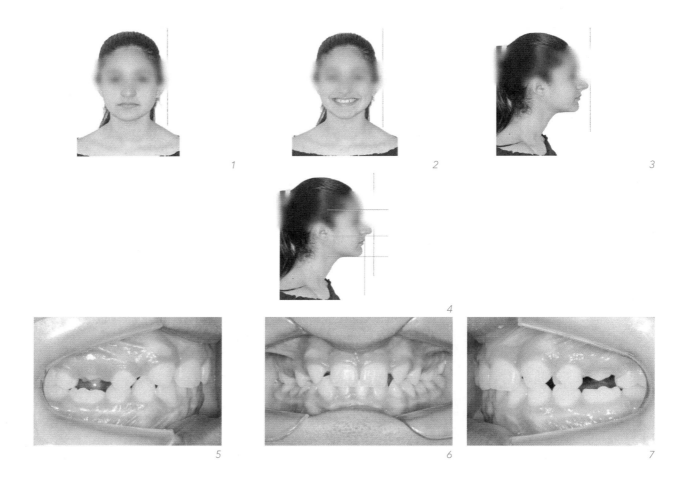

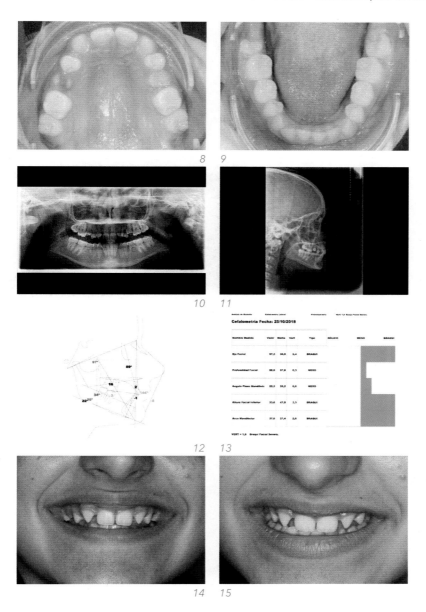

8 9

10 11

12 13

14 15

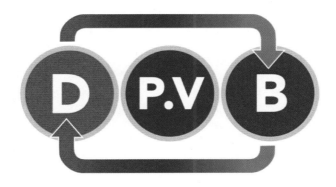

16

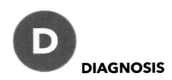 **DIAGNOSIS**

As usual, with our method, let's focus on the diagnosis of her different areas and also on the time-duration of treatment as it is a patient concern because the family is moving abroad.

For the reasons mentioned above, we had 8 months for an essentially aesthetic improvement, which was the main objective of our young patient. *(Fig. 18)*

Age and biotype area

- 13 years' old

- Severe brachyfacial.
  In macro aesthetics, the lower third **(blue)** of the face of the patient was smaller compared to the middle third. *(Figs. 4,11,12 and 13)*

- Nasolabial angle and upper lip curvature are correct. **(green)** *(Fig. 3)*

Dental area. *(Figs. 5 to 10)*

- Increased over bite **(red)**

- Agenesis of teeth # 12, 22 (upper lateral incisors)

- Agenesis of teeth # 35 and 45 (2nd lower premolars)

- Small deviation of the upper midline to left (dental asymmetry)

Functional area

- In maximum intercuspation, she presented a slight mandibular deflection to right (functional asymmetry)

THE MAIN ISSUE

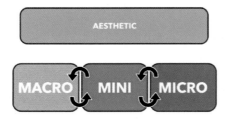

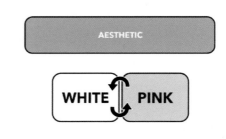

17

18

In these areas we had to especially focus and adopt resolutions on the treatment plan and therapeutic vehicle / s.

We should focus on these areas and adopt resolutions for the treatment plan **P** and therapeutic vehicle(s) **V**.

Based on our experience, we made a list of the aspects that were correct **(green)**, and the aspects to be corrected due to deficit **(blue)** or excess **(red).**

1. There was no full dental mass **(blue)** as there was no complete dental arch. *(Fig. 19).*

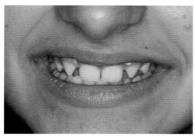

19

2. Good nasolabial angle and volume of the upper lip **(green)**. *(Fig. 20)*

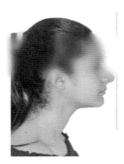

20

3. Logically, the 12-piece smile (blue) did not exist. **(blue)**. *(Fig. 21)*

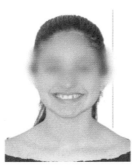

21

4. In the white ⟷ pink aesthetic relationship, at gingival margins level, the aesthetic was far from being minimally acceptable. *(Fig. 22)*

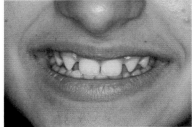

22

5. The ideal 1:0.8 dental ratio showed that the central incisors were "small" in their M-D width. *(Fig. 23)*

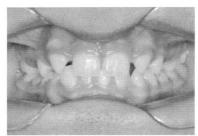

23

6. Due to the absence of teeth # 12 and 22, there were no previous contact areas **(blue)**.

7. There was no smile arc (SAP) *(Fig. 24)*.

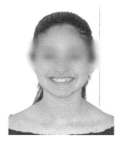

24

8. The vertical display of the central incisors (VID and VIP) was not good.

 TREATMENT PLAN (P)

Future occlusal rehabilitation would involve 2 implants in the areas of agenesis of the lower second

premolars; for age-related reasons, it was not the appropriate time for this procedure and we would only slightly reduce the M-D size of the temporary molars present in the mouth.
Given the agenesis of the upper lateral incisors, there were 2 options, one of them the insertion of implants as a substitute for the missing teeth. *(Fig. 25)*

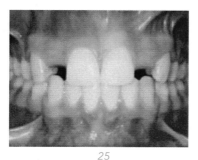

25

This alternative also had the disadvantage of age, but today this can be solved with TADS in the areas of future permanent implants without discomfort and removable or adhered anti-aesthetic prostheses. *(Fig. 26 to 37)*

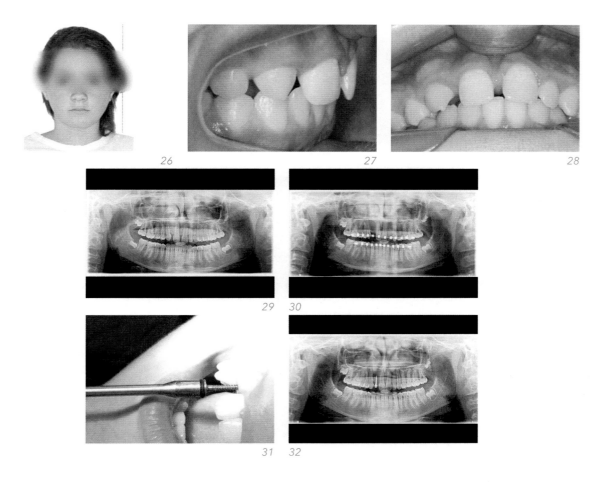

26   27   28

29 30

31 32

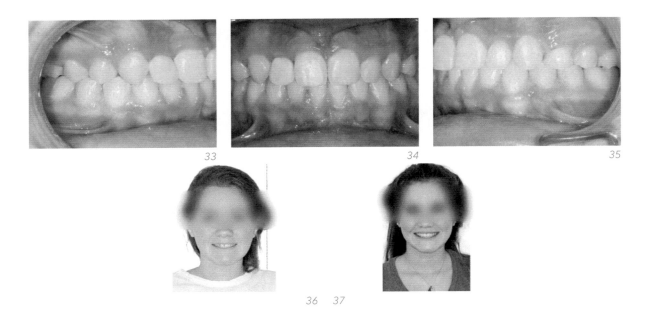

33   34   35

36   37

The other alternative would imply a space adjustment with mesialization of canines, premolars, and molars, changing occlusal and aesthetic roles for various teeth, as can be seen in Figures 33 and 34.

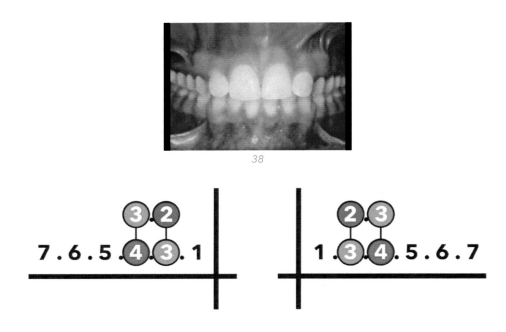

38

39   40

The canines would be lateral incisors, the first premolars would be canines, and the upper molars would occlude in a Class II relationship; the case would also require gingivectomies and morphological changes in some of these teeth.

THERAPEUTIC VEHICLE (V)

Because of the good lip curvature and incisor inclination, we needed a very good 3D control of the anterior superior sector, so, without a doubt, the Pitts21 together with a correct progression of archwires, disarticulations and immediate elastics, would be our therapeutic vehicle, providing us an enormous help, valid for that purpose.

In any case, the brackets and tubes must have a coherent adaptation to the new occlusal scheme proposed in the future.

BIOMECHANICS

1.	BRACKET ADAPTATION
2.	TUBE ADAPTATION IN TEETH # 16 AND 26
3.	ARCHWIRES
4.	FIRST GINGIVECTOMIES AND DENTAL MORPHOLOGICAL CHANGES IN <u>4.3.1</u>|<u>1.3.4</u>
5.	NEW GINGIVECTOMIES AND CHANGES IN DENTAL MORPHOLOGY

88

1 & 2. ADAPTATION OF BRACKETS   AND TUBES IN TEETH # 16 AND 26

Brackets and tubes must be adapted to an aesthetic and occlusal project.

1.	BRACKETS ADAPTATION

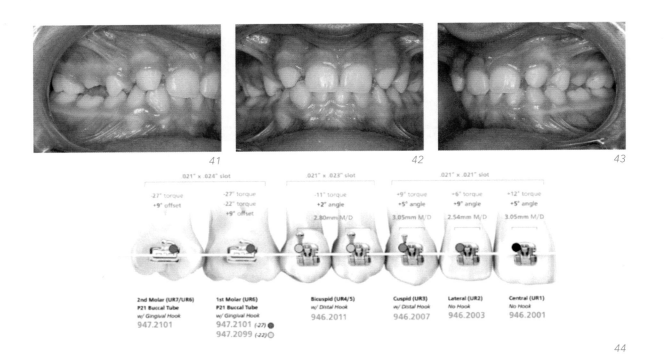

		.021" x .024" slot		.021" x .023" slot		.021" x .021" slot	
-27° torque	-27° torque		-11° torque	+9° torque	+6° torque	+12° torque
+9° offset	-22° torque		+2° angle	+5° angle	+9° angle	+5° angle
	+9° offset		2.80mm M/D	3.05mm M/D	2.54mm M/D	3.05mm M/D

| 2nd Molar (UR7/UR6) P21 Buccal Tube w/ Gingival Hook 947.2101 | 1st Molar (UR6) P21 Buccal Tube w/ Gingival Hook 947.2101 (-27) ● 947.2099 (-22) ○ | Bicuspid (UR4/5) w/ Distal Hook 946.2011 | Cuspid (UR3) w/ Distal Hook 946.2007 | Lateral (UR2) No Hook 946.2003 | Central (UR1) No Hook 946.2001 |

44

The buccal surface of teeth # 13 and 23 was slightly reduced and canine brackets were bonded (with a cut «hook») and with a small error of parallelism to the axis since the upper canine brackets have a 5° angle and those for lateral incisors have 9° (remember teeth # 13 and 23 were going to be # 12 and 22)

We used canine brackets in first premolars, and performed small reduction of their palatal cusps and a first gingivectomy.

The brackets on second premolars, without adjustment, were bonded following a conventional technique.

2. TUBE ADAPTATION IN TEETH # 16 AND 26

When projecting a Class II molar relationship, the upper first molars should be slightly rotated in order to occupy a slightly larger space (approximately 2 mm) in the arch; let's not forget that in these cases half the molar (approx. 5.5 mm) must occupy the M-D space of an entire premolar (approx. 7.5 mm). *(Fig. 45)*

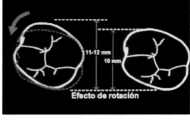

45

To this end, there are 2 solutions:

A. Bond tubes for teeth # 36 and 46 in # 16 and 26. *(Fig. 46)*

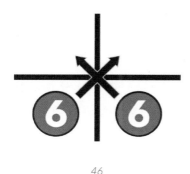

46

We note that the lower right is bonded in the upper left molar and the lower left is also bonded in the opposite and contralateral arch.

The lower tubes have 3° of rotation, while the upper tubes have 9°.

B. The second alternative consists of bonding the upper molar tubes distally to the conventional reference, partially canceling the «offset» degrees. In this patient, we opted for the latter alternative. *(Fig. 47).* H4 tubes (.022 x .026) were bonded in these teeth in order to reduce friction in that area.

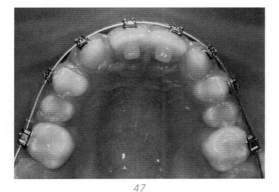

47

3. ARCHWIRES

Because of the time-treatment issues already mentioned, as well as an initial delay in the inclusion of teeth 15 and 25 due to their eruptions, we ended up using only 2 types of archwires in the treatment. *(Figs. 48 to 51)*

.018 x .018 *Niti Ultra Soft Pitts Broad*
.020 x .020 *Niti Pitts Broad*

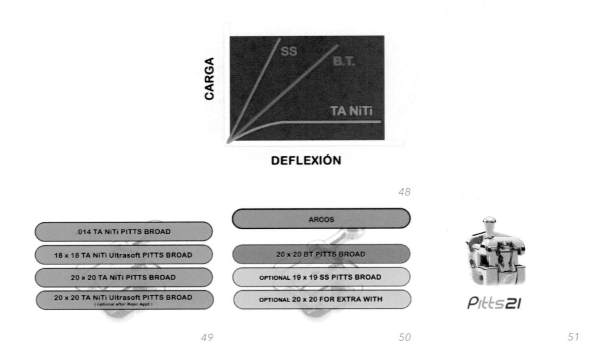

48

.014 TA NiTi PITTS BROAD

18 x 18 TA NiTi Ultrasoft PITTS BROAD

20 x 20 TA NiTi PITTS BROAD

20 x 20 TA NiTi Ultrasoft PITTS BROAD
(optional after Repo Appt)

ARCOS

20 x 20 BT PITTS BROAD

OPTIONAL 19 x 19 SS PITTS BROAD

OPTIONAL 20 x 20 FOR EXTRA WITH

Pitts21

49   50   51

Figures 52 to 57 show the initial treatment with .018 x .018 NiTi Ultra Soft Pitts Broad archwires and 3/16" 2 oz Class III elastics to lose posterosuperior anchorage. Disarticulations and distal displacement are also observable in the bonding of tubes at teeth # 16 and 26.

«Baby eyelets» were bonded in the second temporary molars.

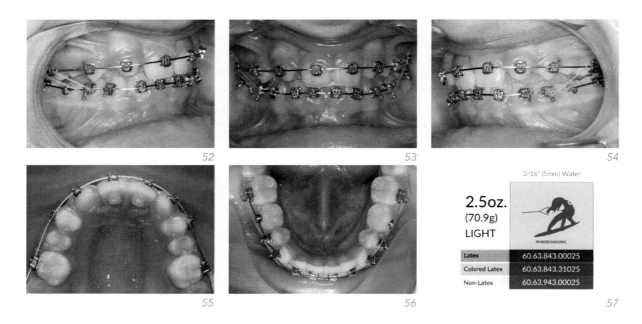

52   53   54

55   56   57

4. FIRST GINGIVECTOMIES AND CHANGES IN DENTAL MORPHOLOGY IN <u>4.3.1|1.3.4</u>

As we entered a bit more into the treatment, we could include the upper second premolars and perform the gingivectomies in canines and central incisors.

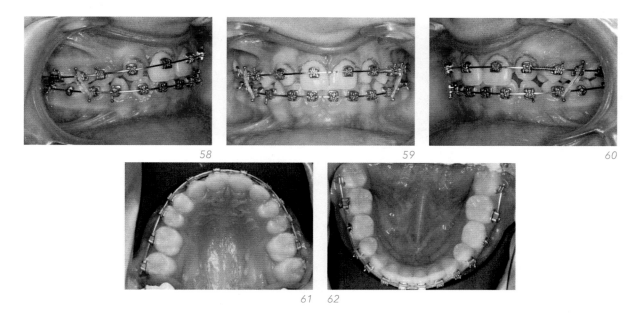

58   59   60

61   62

It is also observable the intention of mesialization of the upper left canine with a NiTi spring with open coils between said tooth and # 24 (which would be 23 in the future occlusal scheme). *(Figs. 58 to 62)*

The following series show the use of NiTi .020 x .020 Pitts Broad archwires in the maxilla and .018 x .018 NiTi Ultra Soft in the mandible. *(Figs. 63 to 66)*

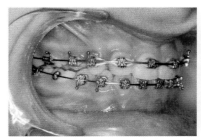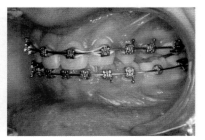

63   64

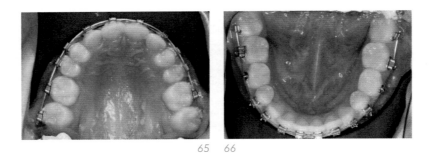

65 66

Photographs 67 to 70 show the final X-rays with the maintenance of good torque in upper incisor.

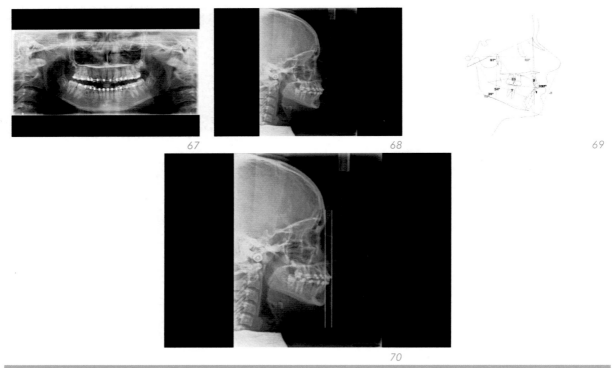

67   68   69

70

5. NEW GINGIVECTOMIES AND CHANGES IN DENTAL MORPHOLOGY

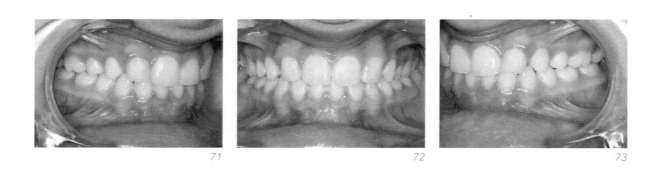

71   72   73

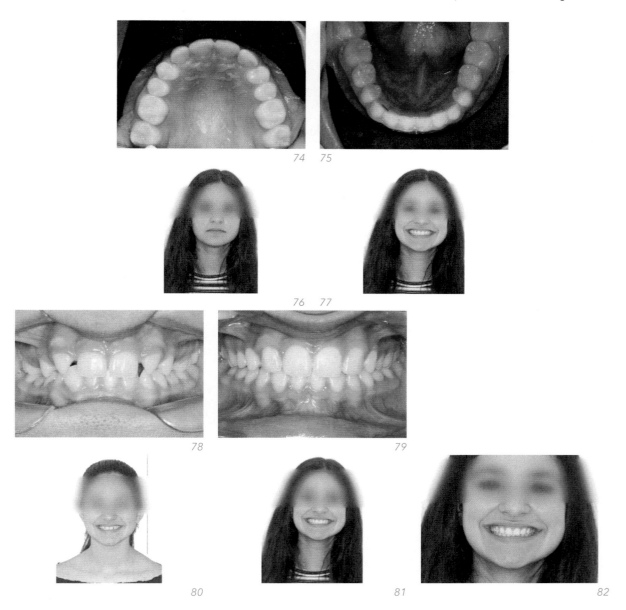

74   75

76   77

78   79

80   81   82

SECTION 4

TIME AND SPACE OF THE 3rd MOLARS

Section 4
Time and Space of the 3rd Molars
Chapter 11
Introduction

You can ask me for anything you want except time.
Napoleon Bonaparte (1769-1840)
Military, French statesman

Orthodontists are prone to carefully assessing the excess and even more so the deficit of space in the anterior sectors of both arches. However, this section aims to make a brief introduction where the assessment of the spaces in the posterior sectors is decisive in the planning or post-treatment of the 2 cases to be discussed.

We will cite some specific studies from the many that have been published which are related to third molars, referring to their development, eruptive path and factors that can affect both the eruption time and the space necessary for their correct positioning in the arches as well as the controversy over their incidence in malpositioned anterior teeth.

The characteristics of the book inhibit any detailed presentation of these studies. We will simply group them in researchers who defend the idea that third molars are the cause of the aforementioned problems, and another group who denies the «pressure from behind theory» as triggering factor for late malpositions in incisor sectors.

First, the introduction of how space and eruption time are related in the distal areas of the second molars. *(Fig 1)*

1. **AGENESIS**

2. **EVOLUTION IN ERUPTION TIME AND SPACE**

3. **SPACE REQUIRED**

4. **INCIDENCE IN INCISOR MALPOSITIONS**

   EXTRACTIONS FOR STABILITY?

5. **FACTORS THAT MODIFY THIRD MOLAR ERUPTION TIME AND SPACE**

6. **EXTRACTIONS FOR TREATMENT?**

1. AGENESIS

Dental agenesis is the absence of one or more teeth. It is a common developmental anomaly in both dentitions, the result of a disorder of the dental lamina, which prevents the formation of dental germ. Any tooth can be absent. The permanent dentition is the most affected. The most frequently absent teeth are the third molars, upper lateral incisors, and lower second premolars.

Third molars are the teeth that occupy the eighth place from the dental median line of each hemiarcade in the permanent dentition, and generally present some anomalous condition such as: variable root morphology (Kuzekanani et al., 2012), eruption problems (Celikoglu et al., 2010; Chu et al., 2003; Hashemipour et al., 2013), congenital absence (Celikoglu et al., 2010; Mok & Ho, 1996; Silva Meza, 2003) and associated pathologies (Celikoglu et al., 2010; Chu et al.) at a lower percentage. Within these conditions, agenesis is a common phenomenon and its prevalence varies.

Researchers place the percentage of agenesis at approximately 10%. *(Figs 2 to 8)*

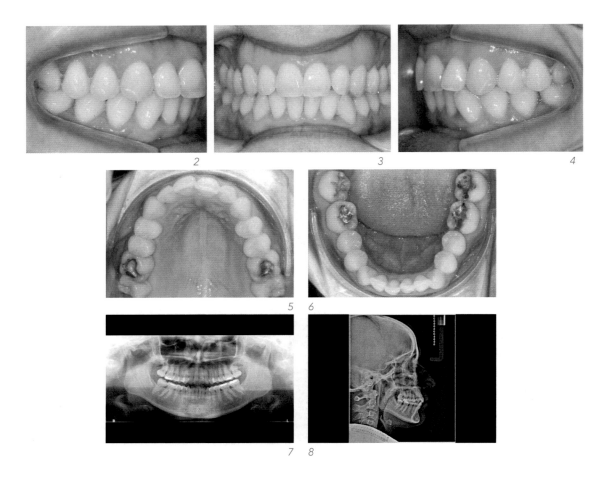

2. EVOLUTION IN ERUPTION TIME AND SPACE

In these and other points we will follow the studies of Dr. Margaret Richardson and Col. (Belfast).

The development of the tooth germ in extremely precocious cases can begin at 5 years and in very late cases at 16, with the maximum percentage of probabilities at 9 years. The crown is completed between the ages of 12 and 18, while the root completion takes place between the ages of 18 and 25.

The average eruption age ranges from between 20 and 24 years. There are factors that have an impact of both the eruption time, as well as in the space available in the mouth.

Dr. Richardson in her work *"The Etiology and Prediction of mandibular third molar impaction"* (1977), investigated the development and eruption path of the lower third molars between individuals 10 and 15 years of age observing that the angle between the occlusal surface of these teeth and the mandibular plane decreased on 11° in average. *(Figs 9 to 13)*

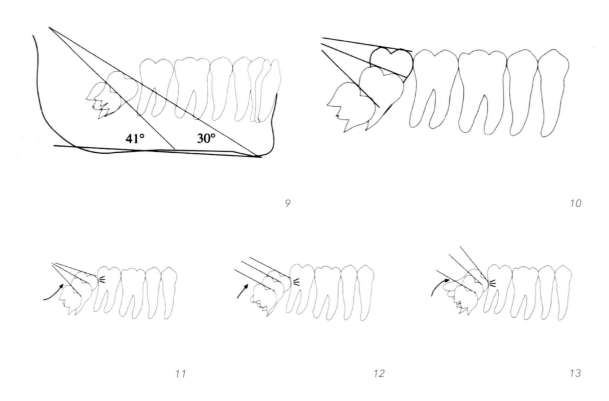

9 10

11 12 13

There are, however, situations of impaction of third molars due to lack of space or at times, unpredictable changes during their eruption path. *(Figs. 14 and 15)*

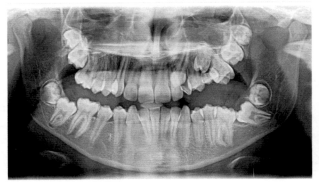
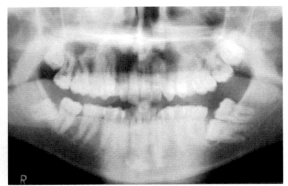

14

15

3. SPACE REQUIRED

While the chances of eruption of the lower wisdom teeth correspond to multiple causes, the main variant is the space or lack thereof and renowned researchers like Drs. Bjork, Ricketts, Graber, among others, have agreed on this topic.

There is an interesting study by Dr. Patrick Turley (1974) that considers that a useful method in evaluating the space available for third molar eruption is the measurement of the distance between mandibular Xi-point and distal surface of mandibular second molars in lateral X-ray.
This work aims to establish a predictive method of eruption using panoramic radiographs to allow us to make the right decision.

This reference is valid for adults, and groups the third molars cases in: retained teeth, erupted in good occlusion and erupted in a bad position; average distances were 21 mm for the first group, 30 mm for the second, and 25 mm for the malpositioned third molars. *(Figs. 16 and 17)*

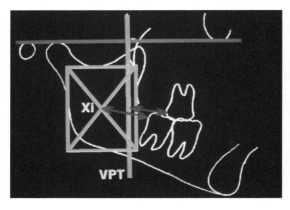
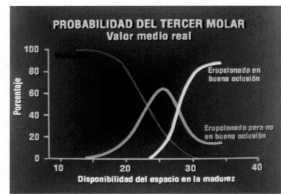

16

17

We reiterate that this study was conducted on adults. In any case "teenage" patients between the ages of 13 and 16 who end the active treatment, would not have a notable increase in growth space in that area either; therefore, with distances less than 25 mm, the possibilities of eruption and correct positioning of the mandibular third molars are almost nil.

4. INCIDENCE IN INCISIVE MALPOSITIONS

It is known that the noticed or expected impaction of the mandible third molars can generate a series of dental problems such as periodontal problems, pericoronitis, occlusal interferences, etc., but what is controversial is whether or not they affect the stability of the incisor sector, especially the mandibular incisor sector.

We are not researchers; we simply present work references with opposing conclusions of the incidence that the postero-anterior pressure of the mandibular third molars would have or would not have. *(Figs. 18 to 23)*

Theory of «Back pressure» - «Pressure from behind theory»			
Vego L. Longitudinal study of mandibular arch perimeter. *Angle Orthod 1962;32:187-92*	Bergstrom K, Jensen R. The significance of third molars in the aetiology of crowding. Trans Europ Soc 1960;36:84-96	Richardson ME. Late lower arch crowding in relation to primary crowding. Angle Orthod 1982;52:300-12	Richardson ME. Lower arch crowding in the young adult.Am J Orthod Dentofac Orthop 1992; 101:132-7
18	*19*	*20*	*21*

Group in disagreement with the incidence of «Back pressure»	
Kaplan RG. Mandibular third molars and postretetion crowding. Am J Orthod 1974; 66:411-30	Sampson WJ, Richards LC, Leigthon BC. Third molar eruption patterns and mandibular dental arch crowding. Aust Orthod J 1983;8:10-20
22	*23*

Our opinion (which is <u>not</u> a research paper), is that there is conflicting evidence on this point and that the causes of inferior malpositions differ individually; they even exist in arches with third molar agenesis, but this does not exclude them as an etiological factor or co-factor in patients who present malpositions as a chief complaint before or after treatment.

Let's not forget 3 variables, which in our opinion, are also important in the genesis of anterior-inferior malpositions.

a. In meso or brachyfacial biotypes, the remnant growth of the mandibular basal area can create this problem.

b. Equalizing premature deflective contacts (upper mesial slopes with lower distal slopes) project the mandible towards a more anterior occlusal comfort positioning with identical results as situation «a».

c. The indication of extractions of mandibular third molars, sooner or later, except in special cases (patient 8), entails a «domino» effect, which bring forth the application of the same procedure in the maxillary molars, which extrude when left without antagonists, resulting in the «b» (equalizer deflective contact) cause.

Many years ago, a patient came for treatment of dental malpositions in both arches, which were especially noticeable in the lower arch.

In her story, she reported having completed a previous treatment to her satisfaction, and that the orthodontist recommended the extraction of third molars.

As can be seen in the Panoramic X-ray, only the mandibular third molars were removed and, consequently, the maxillary third molars extruded, generating an anterior mandibular deflection that also contributed to the lower malpositions even though the third molars of that arch had been removed. *(Figs. 24 to 37)*

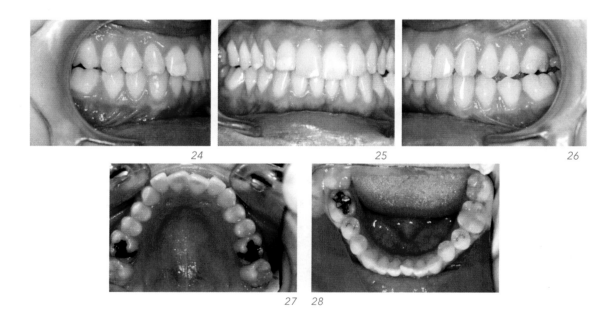

24   25   26

27   28

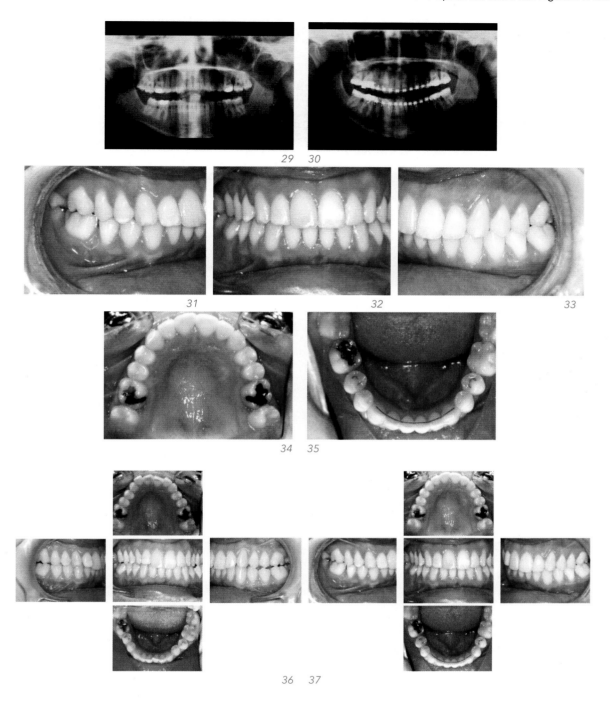

29   30

31   32   33

34   35

36   37

5. FACTORS THAT MODIFY THIRD MOLAR ERUPTION TIME AND SPACE

We have pointed out, and it is known by all that the lack of sufficient space is a factor that affects third molar eruption time and space.

But we will also mention some variables that have an impact on the third molar eruption time and space. *(Fig. 38)*

Space increase
a. Growth
b. Extraction of premolars
c. Extraction of first or second molars

a. Growth

In mandibular growth, there is an increase in the space available for the third molar germs, this also happens in the maxilla. *(Fig. 39)*

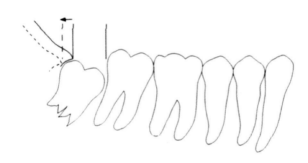

b. Extraction of premolars

The extraction of premolars with a medium anchoring space closure generates, consequently, a variable increase in space for the third molars. *(Fig. 40)*

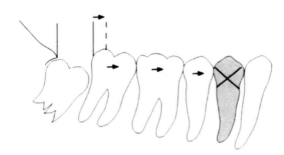

c. Extraction of first or second molars

In this last variable, the extractions in posterior sectors not only increase the space, but also significantly accelerate the average eruption chronology of the third molars; the absence of these posterior teeth, first or second molars, may be a consequence of the dental history of our patient or the result of the treatment plan that we establish. *(Figs. 42 to 60)*

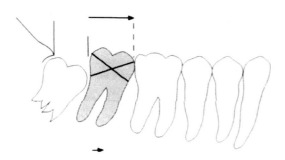

41

19-year-old patient with a dental history of extraction of 36 and 46 (first lower molars).

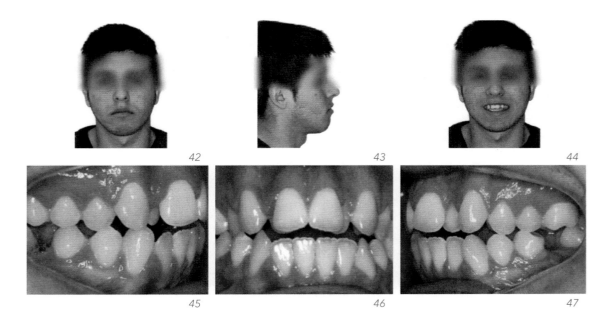

42   *43*   *44*

45   *46*   *47*

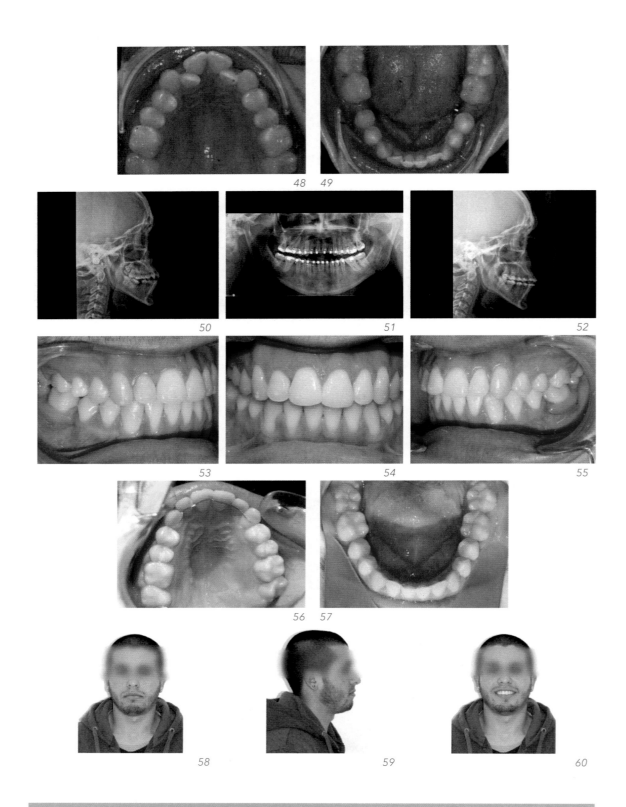

48 49

50 51 52

53 54 55

56 57

58 59 60

6. EXTRACTIONS FOR TREATMENT

We will present images of a case treated some time ago in which the planning consisted of 2 stages; one of them when the patient was 15 years of age, and the second stage at the end patient's growth to provide a small adjustment.

The case was treated some time ago with H4 (.022" x .026" PSL). In this case, both the (P) treatment plan and its biomechanical execution (B) involved the extraction of mandibular second molars which, over time, would be replaced by the development of 2 good third molars germs.

The extraction of teeth # 37 and 47 was to facilitate the vertical (anterior open bite) and anteroposterior (Class III) corrections of the pre-treatment; these corrections were made with simultaneous biomechanics and their protocols (B).

From photograph 61 to 130, we observe the beginning, progression and completion of this treatment stage carried out when the patient was 15 years of age.

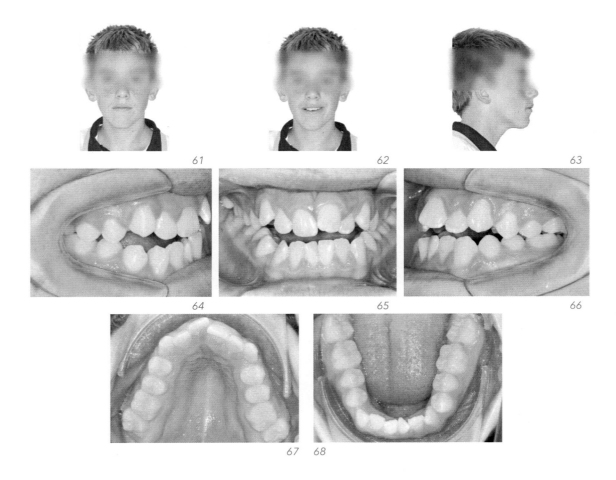

61   62   63

64   65   66

67   68

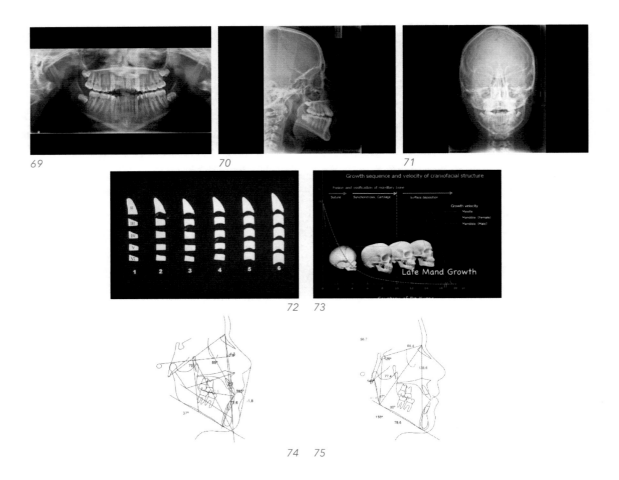

69   70   71

72 73

74 75

The preceding images show a patient in his skeletal age, starting a growth peak that will be unfavorable to correction due to basal and genetic divergence in the mandible.

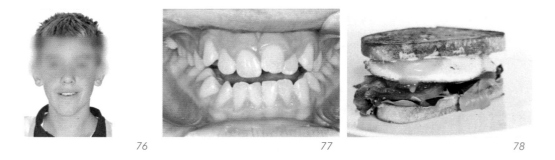

76   77   78

These last 3 images show us the 2 major requirements of the patient in treatment; one to improve dental aesthetic, and two be able to "bite a sandwich" with their anterior teeth.

The case was approached as established, with Simultaneous Biomechanics protocols.

The archwire progression is in accordance with the rectangular slot (.022" x .026") of the H4 brackets and tubes.

Currently, we have further reduced the treatment time and increased the 3D control of the teeth with Pitts21 and its square slot (.021" x.021" in the 3-3 anterior sector) and also square cross-section archwires. *(Fig. 80)*

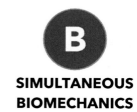

SIMULTANEOUS BIOMECHANICS

Pitts21

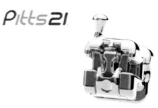

80

– Low friction
– Immediate elastics
– Posterior disarticulations
– Levelled and alignments

– Smile Arc Protection (SAP)
– Vertical Incisor Display (VID)
– Arch Development

82

– Cross correction
– Vertical correction
– Anteroposterior correction

83

– Lingual re-education (Lingual reminders + «lifting» exercises)

84

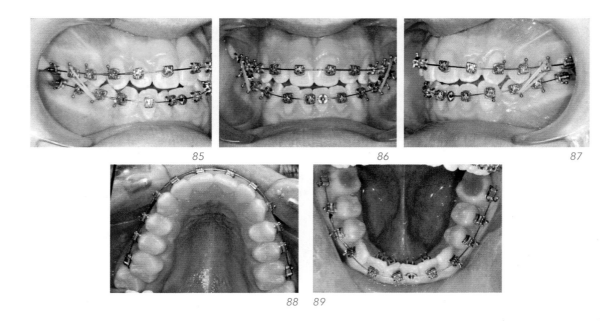

85   86   87

88 89

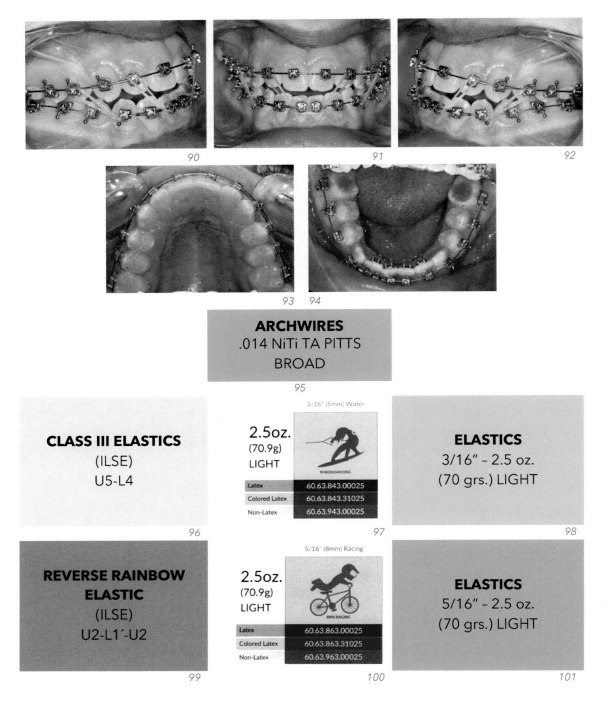

ARCHWIRES
.014 NiTi TA PITTS
BROAD

95

CLASS III ELASTICS
(ILSE)
U5-L4

96

3/16" (5mm) Water

2.5oz.
(70.9g)
LIGHT

WAKEBOARDING

Latex	60.63.843.00025
Colored Latex	60.63.843.31025
Non-Latex	60.63.943.00025

97

ELASTICS
3/16" – 2.5 oz.
(70 grs.) LIGHT

98

REVERSE RAINBOW ELASTIC
(ILSE)
U2-L1´-U2

99

5/16" (8mm) Racing

2.5oz.
(70.9g)
LIGHT

BMX RACING

Latex	60.63.863.00025
Colored Latex	60.63.863.31025
Non-Latex	60.63.963.00025

100

ELASTICS
5/16" – 2.5 oz.
(70 grs.) LIGHT

101

We used .018" x .018" *NiTi Ultrasoft Pitts Broad* archwire for the first time, which qualities are now noticeably enhanced with Pitts21 brackets. *(Figs. 102 to 104)*

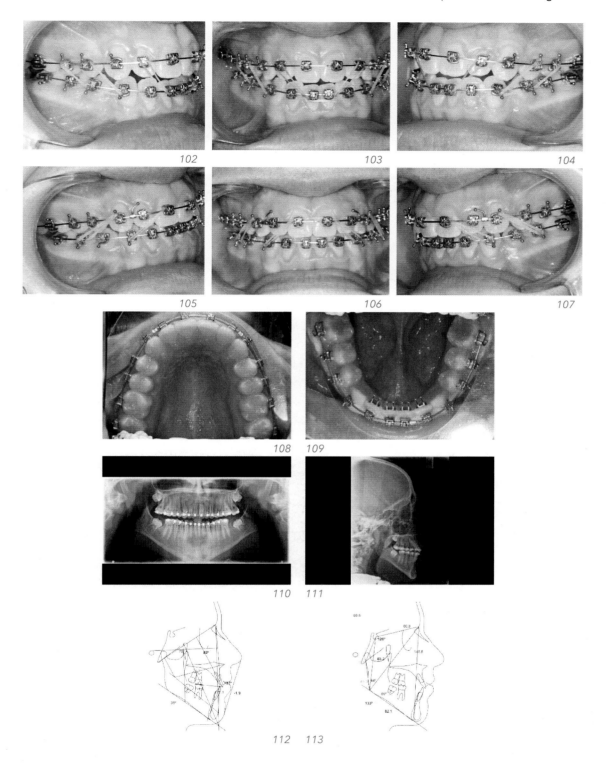

102 *103* *104*

105 *106* *107*

108 *109*

110 *111*

112 *113*

Before moving to .016" x .025" and .018 x.025" NiTi Pitts Broad archwires, .018 x .025" archwires made of Beta Titanium were used. *(Figs 105 to 109)*

Figs. 110 to 128 show dental and facial X-rays at the end of this treatment that, we repeat, will have an adjustment 4 years later at the end of the patient's growth.

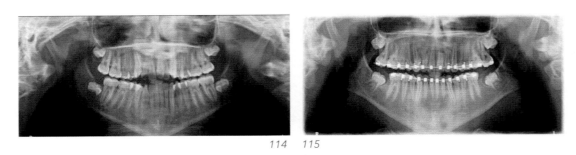

114   115

The main objectives were to satisfy the patient requirements and to try to change his epigenetics.

The genetic influences on the development of Class III malocclusion include hereditary effects on both the masticatory muscles and the mandibular skeletal morphology. However, beyond genetic variations, the characteristics of muscles and bones are also influenced by epigenetic mechanisms that produce differences in the gene expression. (Huh A, Horton MJ, Cuenco KT, et al. Epigenetic influence of KAT6B and HDAC4 in the development of skeletal malocclusion).

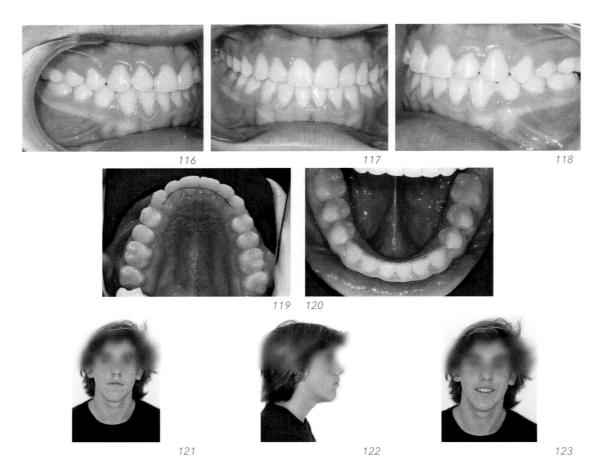

116   117   118

119   120

121   122   123

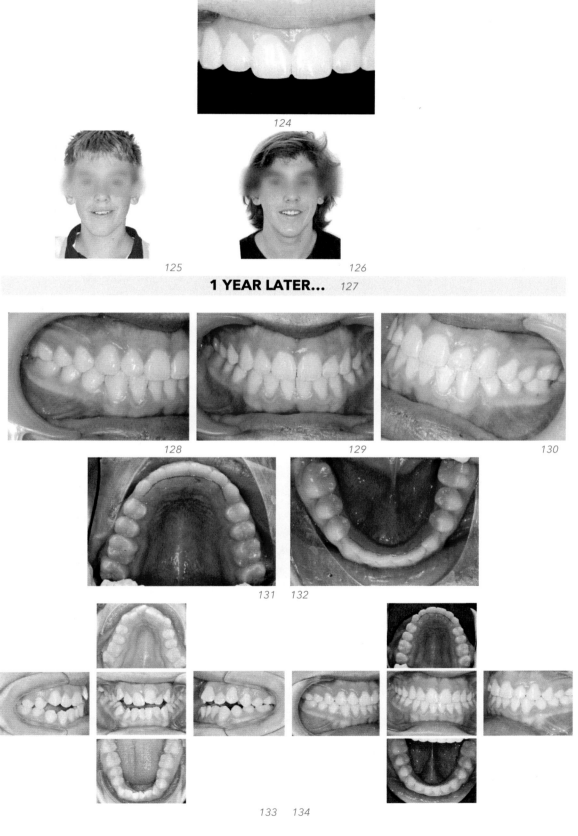

124

125 126

1 YEAR LATER... 127

128 129 130

131 132

133 134

The following 4 figures show the evolution of third molar germs from pre-treatment, end of active treatment, and 1 year and 3 years after treatment, respectively.

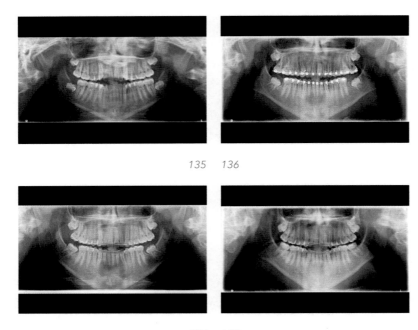

135 136

137 138

However, beyond this last case, it is convenient to go back to the fact that there are extractions of third molars that are part of the treatment (P) plan and almost of the (B) biomechanics, as occurs in open bites of divergent patients. *See patients 4 and 8*

Don't give up,
you still have time
to reach up and start anew;
accept your shadows,
bury your fears,
free your burdens,
fly again.

Mario Benedetti (1920-2009)
Uruguayan writer and poet.

Section 4
Time and Space of the 3rd Molars
Chapter 12
Patient 7

I wasted time, now time doth waste me.
William Shakespeare, (1564-1616)
English playwright, poet and actor.

There are cases that can perfectly be placed in any of the previous sections since they have links with Aesthetics, Simultaneous Biomechanics, Asymmetries, Third Molars, Eruption Time and Space.

This was the case of a patient who deserves to be in this book because she believed in us, because she collaborated enormously in the multidisciplinary treatment and because her story had a happy ending.

A few years ago, we were in our office when a new patient arrived… She was thin, black hair, just an ordinary 14-year-old teenager... But what most caught our attention was that she was afraid to smile. She didn't like to do it, and would avoid it entirely.

The fundamental treatment requirements of this 14-year-old patient were related to the aesthetic of her upper teeth.

Another major concern was that, due to the existence of a bone defect in the maxillary interincisal mid-sector, previous clinicians told her that the possibility of orthodontics was not available to her because if treatment was carried out she was told extraction of teeth # 14 and 24 was necessary.

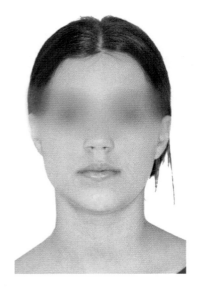 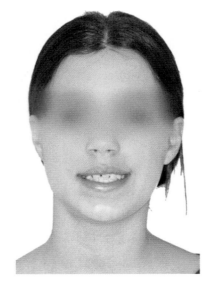

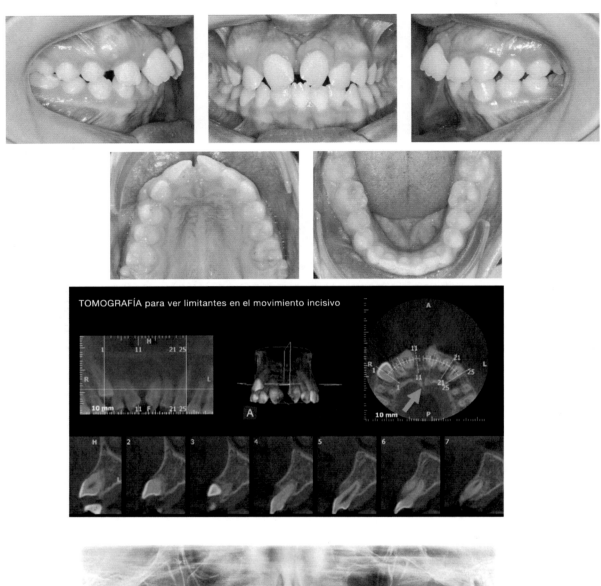

TOMOGRAFÍA para ver limitantes en el movimiento incisivo

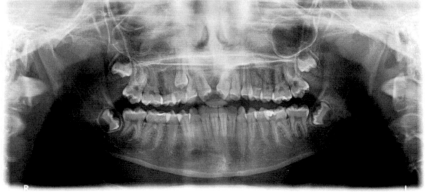

After showing her extra and intraoral images as well as the panoramic X-ray and her computed tomography, we will begin to implement and describe "our DPVB method", step by step.

Starting with the DIAGNOSIS:

DPVB METHOD

D DIAGNOSIS

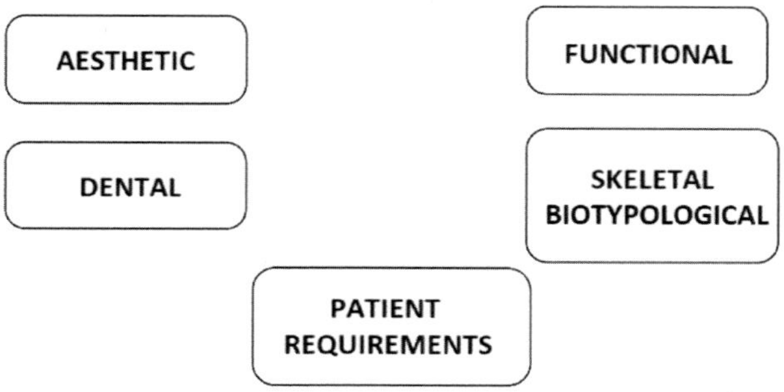

AESTHETIC

FUNCTIONAL

DENTAL

SKELETAL BIOTYPOLOGICAL

PATIENT REQUIREMENTS

From the diagnostic point of view, we are going to consider 5 factors:

1. **AESTHETIC**

2. **DENTAL**

3. **FUNCTIONAL**

4. **SKELETAL / BIOTYPOLOGICAL**

5. **PATIENT REQUIREMENTS**

Aesthetic analysis and patient requirements

Regarding these diagnostic factors, as we mentioned at the beginning of this chapter, 9 out of 10 patients will have aesthetics as their main requirement. Dr. Sarver classifies the aesthetic analysis, and divides it into 3:

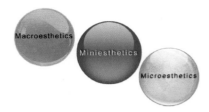

- **MACROAESTHETICS**

- **MINIAESTHETICS**

- **MICROAESTHETICS**

For practical purposes, and to continue simplifying the daily work at the clinic, we recommend that you make this diagnosis in a visual way as Dr. Dwight Frey does by assigning colors (diagnostic visualization) and NOT by using numbers or cephalometric values that can be hard to remember later.

- As we mentioned in the first section of the book

Dr. Dwight Frey performs this assessment using 3 colors to which we add the yellow color, considering the time as a determining factor for certain modifications.

DIAGNOSTIC VISUALIZATION BASED ON 4 COLORS

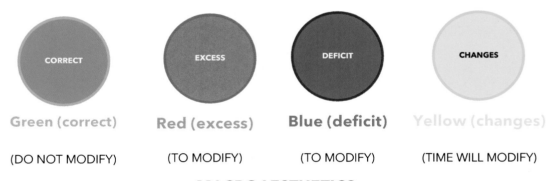

Green (correct)	Red (excess)	Blue (deficit)	Yellow (changes)
(DO NOT MODIFY)	(TO MODIFY)	(TO MODIFY)	(TIME WILL MODIFY)

MACROAESTHETICS

- VERTICAL PROPORTIONS
- HORIZONTAL PROPORTIONS
- LIP CLOSURE

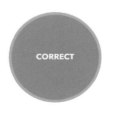

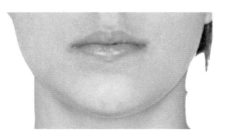

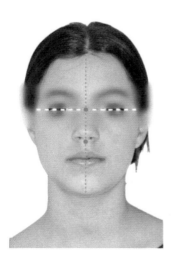

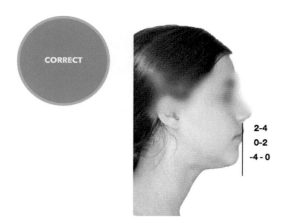

- NASOLABIAL ANGLE
- NASAL PROJECTION
  (NASAL TIP)
- PROFILE

In **MACROAESTHETICS,** in the frontal view, we have to take into account:

- VERTICAL PROPORTIONS
- HORIZONTAL PROPORTIONS
- LIP CLOSURE

And, on the *lateral or profile view*, we have to take into account:

- Nasolabial angle
- Mentolabial angle
- Nasal projection (Nasal tip)
- Upper lip, lower lip and chin projection. Ideal aesthetic proportions in the adult and with respect to the projected subnasal vertical line.

Taking all this into account all this for clinical simplification and its eventual diagnostic visualization, we will assign the green color which means "**DO NOT MODIFY"** since it is correct.

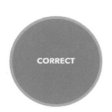

DIGITAL OVERLAY OF IMAGES

This digital overlay of images is simply done for practical purposes and to verify FACIAL SYMMETRY.

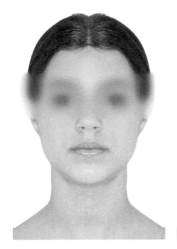 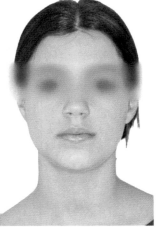 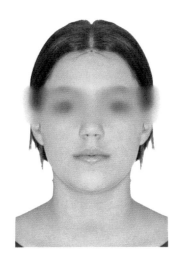

RIGHT HALVES   ORIGINAL   LEFT HALVES

MINIAESTHETICS

- VISUALIZATION OF INCISORS

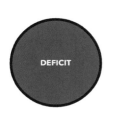

SAP

VIP

VID

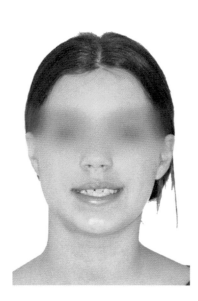

- BUCCAL CORRIDORS

- GINGIVAL DISPLAY

- SMILE HEIGHT

In **MINIAESTHETICS**, we have to take into account:

- VISUALIZATION OF INCISORS AND RELATED TO SAP, VIP AND VID.

- FACIAL MIDLINE.

- BUCCAL CORRIDORS.

- • GINGIVAL DISPLAY.

- We see that the majority of aspects related to mini-aesthetics are in deficit and we assign them the **BLUE** color (TO MODIFY).

- Visualization of incisors in **BLUE**, taking into account the "**today**" status of the patient as there are age-related changes that would aggravate the current situation as shown in the table.

AVERAGE DENTAL DISPLAY AT REST (MM)[7]		
	Maxillary Central Incisor	Mandibular Central Incisor
Less than 30	**3.4**	**0.5**
30 - 40	**1.6**	**0.8**
40 - 50	**1.0**	**2.0**
50 - 60	**0.5**	**2.5**
More than 60	**0.0**	**3.0**

In sum, SAP (**S**mile **A**rc **P**rotection), VIP (**V**ertical **I**ncisor **P**osition) and VID (**V**ertical **I**ncisor **D**isplay), which play a fundamental role in mini-aesthetics, were in deficit..

MICROAESTHETICS

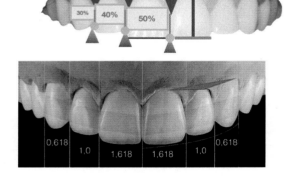

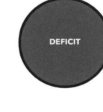

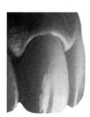

INDIVIDUAL

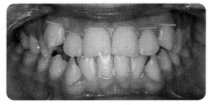

by GROUP

- • RELATED FACTORS

- • DENTAL ANALYSIS

When we analyze **MICROAESTHETICS**; we have to consider that it is a dental assessment and analysis, both individually and as a whole.

- At this point, all factors related to MAINTAINING or MODIFYING proportions of white aesthetic (tooth) and pink aesthetic (gingiva) will be important.

- Here we clearly see a **DEFICIT** in that aspect.

DENTAL ANALYSIS

In the frontal view, we observe a dentoalveolar narrowing, caused by a functional imbalance, both of the upper arch and lower arch, forming what we call the HOURGLASS in the dentoalveolar area.

We also observe some anterior proinclination.

A **dental asymmetry** is observed, with a right deviation of the maxillary midline caused by the retention of tooth # 1.3.

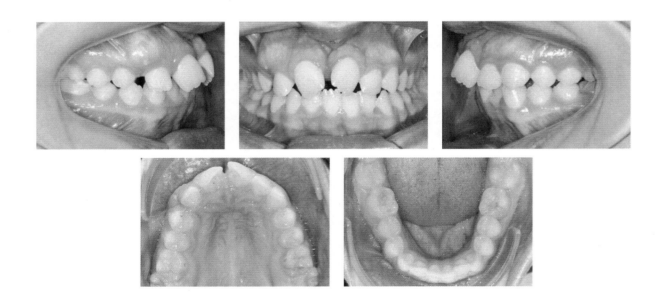

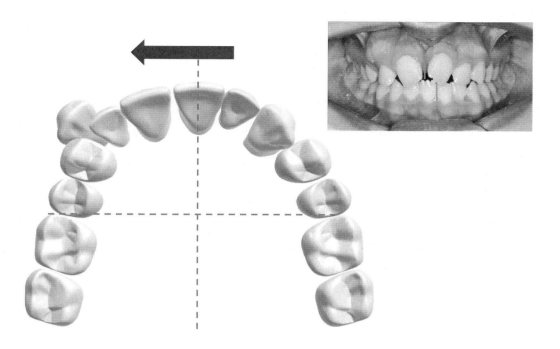

The most frequent dental retentions, according to Peterson [1], are the third molars and permanent canines.

Lower·third·molar	35%
Upper·canine	34%
Upper·third·molar	9 %
Lower·second·premolar	5 %
Lower·canine	4 %
Lower·central·incisor	4 %
Upper·second·premolar	3 %
Lower·first·premolar	2 %
Upper·lateral·incisor	1.5%

[1] Peterson L J 1998. Principles of management of impacted teeth. In Peterson L J, Ellis E, Hupp J R, Tucker M R (eds) Contemporary oral and maxillofacial surgery. Mosby, St. Louis, pp. 215-248.

The lateral view shows a Class II canine relationship.

The upper and lower occlusal views show the existing negative discrepancy in the arches and the dental asymmetry blocking tooth # 1.3.

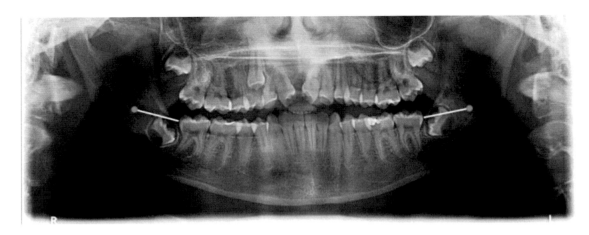

• Punto Xi

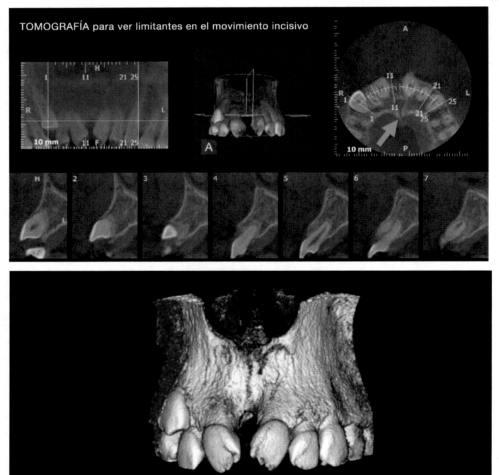

After analyzing the panoramic X-ray and Tomography, we observe:

- Retention of tooth # 1.3.

- The existence of a bone defect in the maxillary interincisal mid-sector was a factor to consider in the planning, execution, stability and health of the dental movement to be carried out.

- Mandibular third molars WITHOUT SPACE for correct eruption (distance from distal side to Xi-point of 22mm)

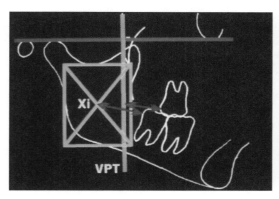 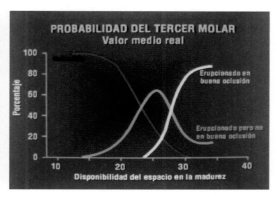

PLANNING AND THERAPEUTIC VEHICLES (PV)

The factors listed in the previous point make us think that we are facing a case for extraction of premolars.

This is where we ask ourselves the big question: "Does the tooth move WITH the bone or THROUGH the bone?"

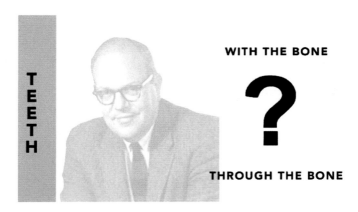

At all times, it was taken into account that it would be a multidisciplinary treatment due to the aforementioned bone defect and to the fact that it was essential to act with biologically suitable and soft forces that, at the same time, achieve the development of the arches, good rotational correction and torque expression in order to **move the teeth with the bone and not through the bone**.

As a therapeutic vehicle, we chose the passive self-ligating, initially with the H4 bracket (0.22 x .026" slot) and after 4 months, they were switched to Pitts21 brackets (021 x .021" slot) in the anterior-superior and anterior-inferior sectors

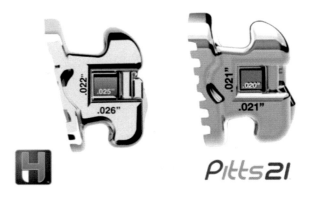

B

SIMULTANEOUS BIOMECHANICS

The Biomechanics part of the treatment is ALWAYS carried out by taking into account these concepts of simultaneous biomechanics *(See section 2)*.

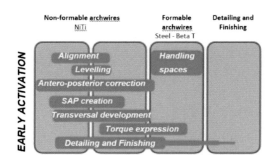

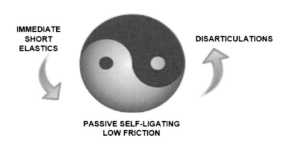

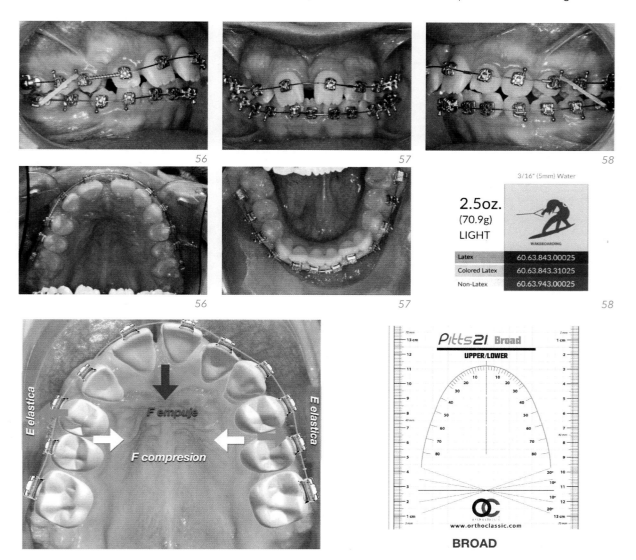

TRANSVERSAL DEVELOPMENT WITH PITTS BROAD IS KEY TO THE CORRECTION OF THE ANTERIOR SECTOR

Short Class II elastics, 3/16" diameter, 2.5 oz. force were also used.
To remember, the disarticulations pursue the following objectives:

OBJECTIVES	• TO ENHANCE THE ARCHWIRE ACTION • (INTRA ARCH)
	• TO ENHANCE THE ELASTIC ACTION • (INTER ARCH)
	• TO APPLY A SELECTIVE VERTICAL CONTROL • (OPEN BITE - DEEP BITE)

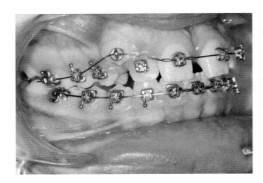
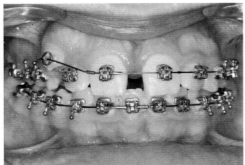

Passing the .014" NiTi Pitts Broad archwire in the arch WITHOUT the connection of all teeth, and also increasing the inter-bracket distance were performed to lower the load-deflection ratio, and to not cause the anterior binding.

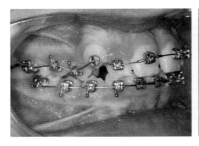
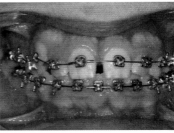
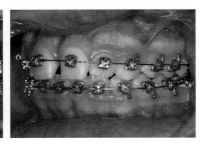

The .014" NiTi Pitts Broad archwire connected all teeth when the angle of incidence was not such, so as to cause binding.

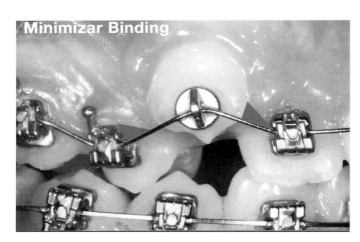

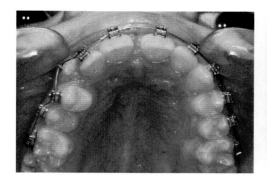
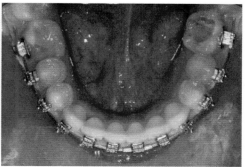

Then, the aforementioned changes to Pitts 21 brackets were made, which with its association with square cross-section archwires allow us a 3D control (TIP TORQUE and ROTATION) of the teeth and a decrease of 30-40% in the forces exerted on.

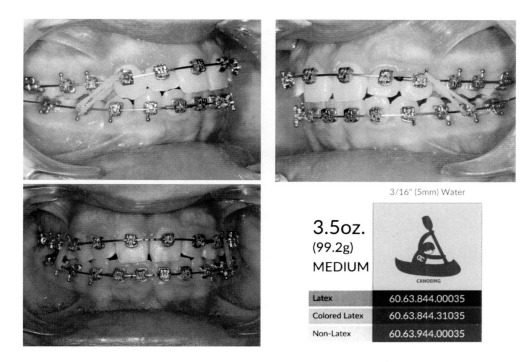

Two months later, .020 x .020" NiTi Pitts Broad were installed and the elastics were changed to 3.5 oz.

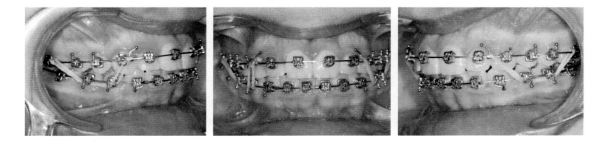

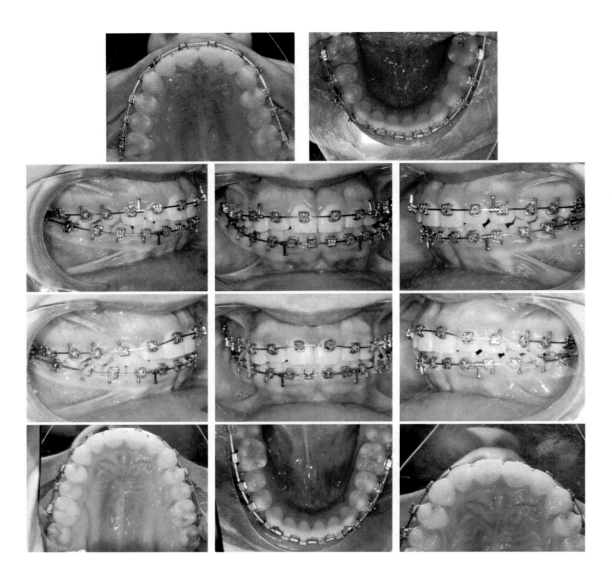

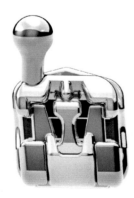

Pitts21

Pitts 21 Full Sequence

∩ .014 TA NiTi Pitts Broad

∩ 18x18 TA NiTi UltraSoft Pitts Broad
(starting point if crowding is mild)

∩ 20x20 TA NiTi Pitts Broad

∩ 20x20 TA NiTi Ultrasoft Pitts Broad
(optional after Repo Appt)

∩ 20x20 BT Pitts Broad

∩ Optional 19x19 SS Pitts Broad for Extraction cases
Optional 20x20 SS for Extra Width

Then, .019 x .019" steel archwires were used in an individual and inter-coordinated way.

Therefore, so far, our sequence of Pitts21 archwires was the following, considering that the .014" NiTi Pitts Broad was the first archwire used in the H4 bracket.

Finally, the brackets were recommended for the upper incisors to improve the SAP (smile arch protection) and VID (vertical incisor display). For this, .0.18 x .018" NiTi Ultra Soft archwires were used again, and, 40 days later, they were changed to .020 x .020" NiTi Pitts Broad.

After these movements, Dr. Walter Ferro (Maxillary Surgeon) performed bone grafting and membrane placing in the upper interincisor sector.

The archwires and brackets were kept unchanged and a 5-month-period passed, waiting for the bone regeneration of the area, which is noticeable in the panoramic X-ray.

GUIDED BONE REGENERATION FOR POST-TREATMENT STABILITY

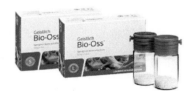

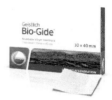

Synthetic bone of bovine origin   Resorbable collagen membrane

POST TREATMENT

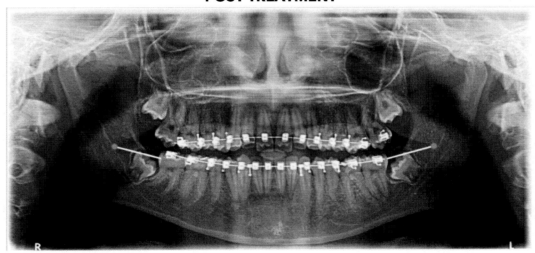

This final Panoramic X-ray also corroborates what we had diagnosed in the initial X-ray regarding the position of the mandibular third molars, the measurements showed us that they DID NOT HAVE SPACE for a correct eruption (from the distal side of molar # 7 to Xi-point 22 mm).

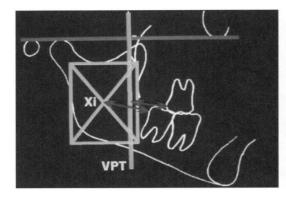

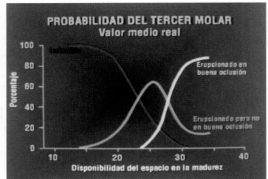

PRE TREATMENT **POST TREATMENT**

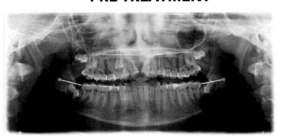

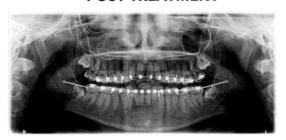

• Punto Xi

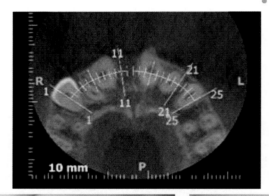

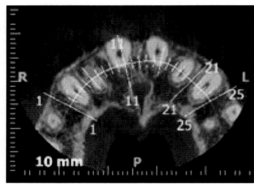

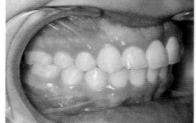

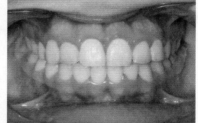

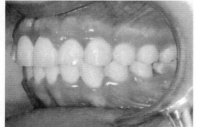

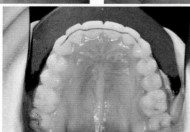

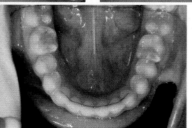

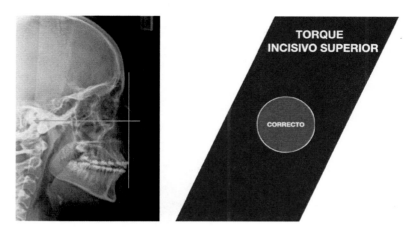

In the lateral X-ray, we observe the patient's correct final torque.

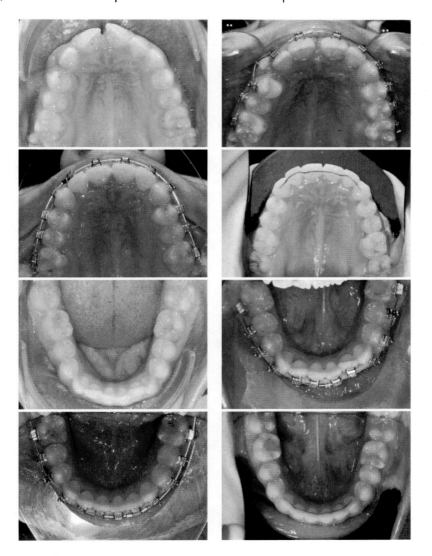

Comparison of the development of the upper and lower arches in the progression of archwires.

MICROAESTHETICS

INITIAL

FINAL

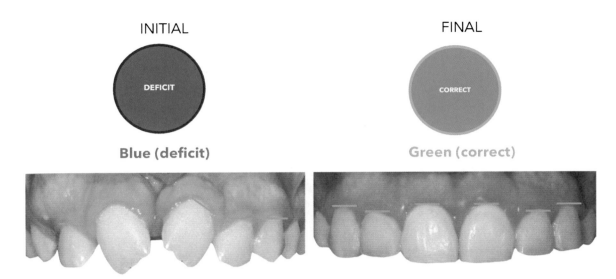

DEFICIT

CORRECT

Blue (deficit)

Green (correct)

COMPARISON OF MICROAESTHETICS

MINIAESTHETICS

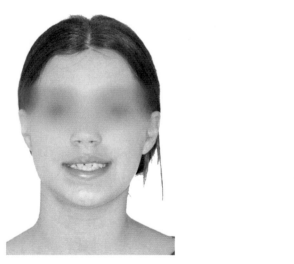

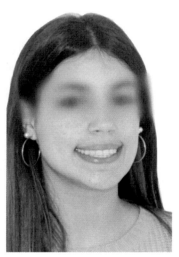

COMPARISON OF MINIAESTHETICS

Section 4
Time and Space of the 3rd Molars
Chapter 13
Patient 8

Many cases that come to our dental office have, among themselves, similarities, but above all variants that make them unique.

No one is like another, neither better nor worse, it is another,
and if two agree it is because of a misunderstanding.
Jean Paul Sartre (1905-1980)
Writer and existentialist philosopher.

This patient (#8) has similarities with the cases presented in the second and third sections, but, at the same time, certain peculiarities that justify its analysis and, to a great extent, the Biomechanics **B** used.

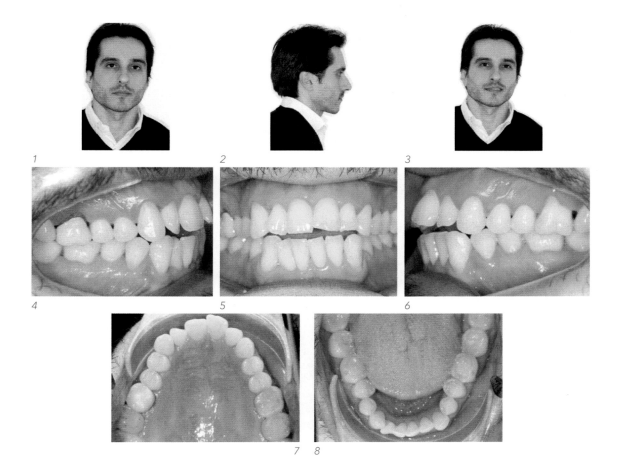

1   2   3

4   5   6

7   8

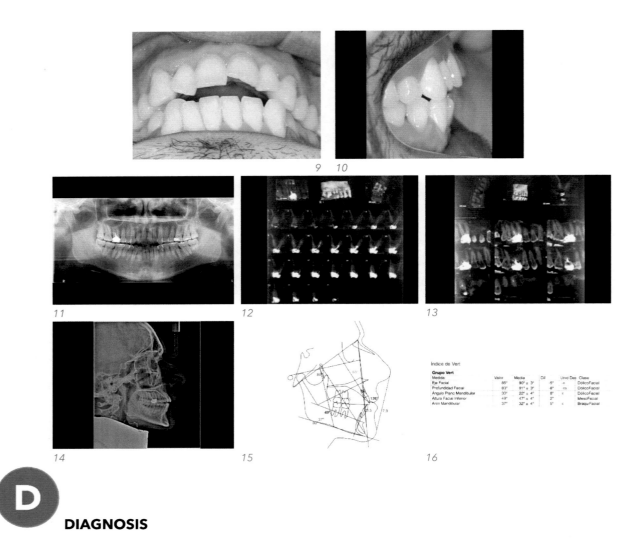

9 10

11 12 13

14 15 16

D DIAGNOSIS

From Figures 1 to 16, we expose the main images of the pre-treatment and some of them will be later detailed.

The incisive malpositions, especially the superior incisors, (mini-aesthetic) along with occlusal functional problems related to difficulties in cutting food in the anterior sector were the reasons for consultation; the time-duration factor of treatment was not a patient's requirement. *(Figs. 17 and 18)*

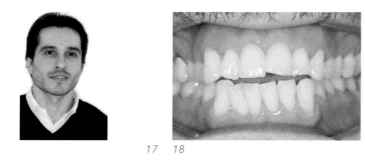

17 18

Analyzing the macro-aesthetic-biotype relation relationship, we noticed in the facial thirds, a certain predominance of the lower third over the middle third, which is consistent with a posterior rotational trend (mild dolycho - in biotype). *(Figs 19 to 22)*

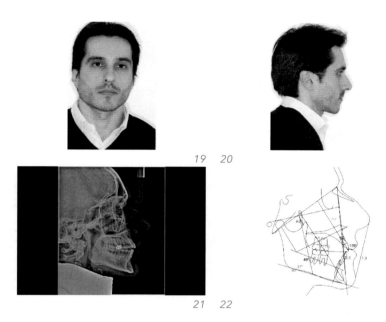

19   20

21   22

In the dental area there were fundamental elements to design the Treatment Plan; at occlusal level, there was poor transverse coordination between arches, with open bite and anterior malpositions that caused a reverse curve of smile. The anteroposterior showed a Class I relationship with the presence of third molars in the mouth, and clinically and radiographically significant periodontal problem was noted, especially in the lower incisor-canine sectors and the upper left first molar. *(Figs 23 a 29)*

Tooth 16 offered, according to its treating dentist, almost zero chances of successful treatment for its permanence in the mouth.

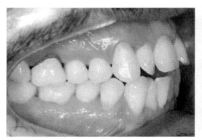 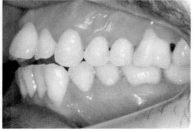

23   24

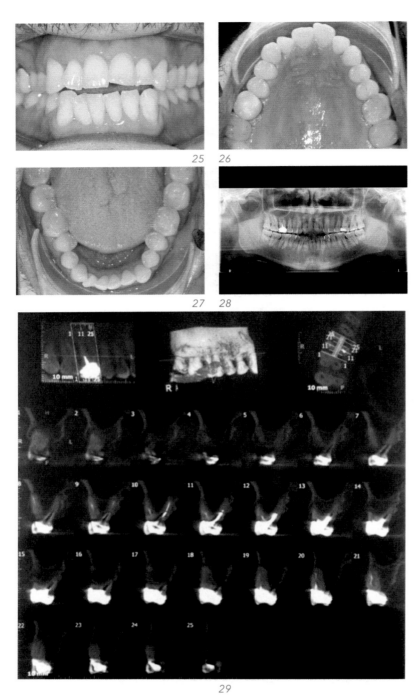

25 26

27 28

29

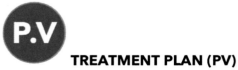

TREATMENT PLAN (PV)

When designing the treatment plan **P**, we started with the assumption that piece 16 was in good health. In this theoretical scenario, we would indicate the extraction of the 4 third molars as it is a case of a divergent (dolycho) patient with an anterior open bite.

To this first decision we would add the simultaneous biomechanics, Pitts21 (PSL), anterior elastics (ILSE), posterior disarticulations, adequate archwire progression, smile arch design (SAP), we would facilitate the correct vertical exposure of upper incisors (VIP) and would recommend neuromuscular exercise; the duration of active treatment was estimated to be between 8 and 9 months.

But the cases are as they are, and the upper right first molar was condemned to extraction, so we presented the patient with 2 different options.
1) Extraction of third molars and tooth # 16, and it with an implant.

   Duration of treatment 8 to 9 months.
2) Extraction of # 28 - 38 - 48 and 16, closure of gaps with minimal anchoring biomechanics where the 2nd and 3rd molars of the upper right quadrant are mesialized and replace the 1st and 2nd molars, respectively.

This last plan did not include an implant, but it needed approximately 5 more months of active treatment. Even with the aforementioned simultaneous biomechanics.
Patient 8 chose this last option, which in opinion was correct. *(Fig. 30)*

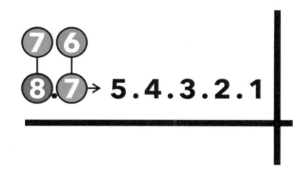

30

THERAPEUTIC VEHICLES (PV)

As vehicles , Pitts21brackets were to be used with posterior disarticulations, and elastics (ILSE), and adequate progression of arches, NiTi spring with closed coils with eyelets and lingual reminders. *(Fig. 31 A 38)*

In biomechanics **B** we will examine the tubes used in teeth # 18 and 17.

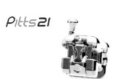

Pitts21

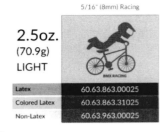

5/16" (8mm) Racing

2.5oz.
(70.9g)
LIGHT

Latex	60.63.863.00025
Colored Latex	60.63.863.31025
Non-Latex	60.63.963.00025

31   32

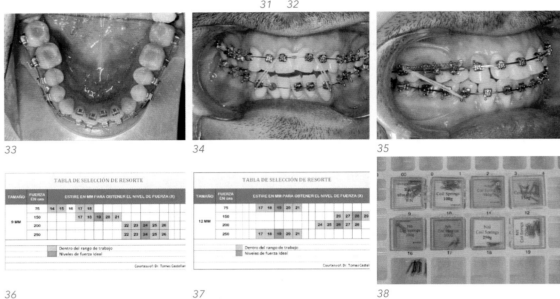

33

34

35

TABLA DE SELECCIÓN DE RESORTE

TAMAÑO	FUERZA EN grs	ESTIRE EN MM PARA OBTENER EL NIVEL DE FUERZA (X)											
9 MM	75	14	15	16	17	18							
	150				17	18	19	20	21				
	200								22	23	24	25	26
	250								22	23	24	25	26

Dentro del rango de trabajo
Niveles de fuerza ideal

Courtesy of: Dr. Tomas Castellan

36

TABLA DE SELECCIÓN DE RESORTE

TAMAÑO	FUERZA EN grs	ESTIRE EN MM PARA OBTENER EL NIVEL DE FUERZA (X)											
12 MM	75		17	18	19	20	21						
	150							26	27	28	29		
	200							24	25	26	27	28	
	250		17	18	19	20	21						

Dentro del rango de trabajo
Niveles de fuerza ideal

Courtesy of: Dr. Tomas Castel

37

38

B

SIMULTANEOUS BIOMECHANICS

Having defined the (D) diagnosis and established a (P) treatment plan which involved, among other objectives, a tooth movement towards the mesial surface of teeth # 17 and 18, the (B) biomechanics were established, many of them happening concurrently in time and according to the chosen (V) vehicles.

1) Space closure.

2) Tubes in teeth # 18 and 17.

3) Archwire progression.

4) Disarticulations.

5) Elastics.

6) Springs.

7) Neuromuscular exercise.

1. Space closure

After the extraction of tooth # 16, we should perform the closure of a large space (approximately 11 mm) with a movement called minimum anchorage, that is, the mesial movement of the second and third upper molars.

Let's remember the biomechanical factors for the handling and implementation when closing large spaces. *(Fig. 39)*

1. **VALUE OF DENTAL UNITS**
2. **SELECTIVE FRICTION**
3. **"COMBINATION" OF FORCES**
4. **LIMITING BIOLOGICAL FACTORS**
5. **TADS POSSIBILITIES**
6. **POSTERIOR SPACES**

39

2. Tubes in # 18 and 17

Assuming that Pitts21 and its adequate biomechanics were the best therapeutic vehicle, we should examine its progressive bracket slot since we were interested in using factor n° 2 (selective friction) for closing the space of tooth # 16. As seen in figures 40 to 45, the slot of Pitts21 molar tubes is .021 x .024, so we decided to change them to H4 tubes that are .022 x .026 to reduce the friction of the right posterior sector and thus facilitate its mesial movement.

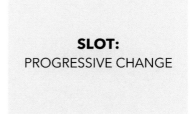

SLOT:
PROGRESSIVE CHANGE

40

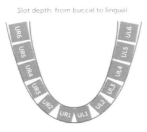

Slot depth, from buccal to lingual

41

SQUARE
FOR ANTERIOR SECTORS
RECTANGULAR
FOR POSTERIOR SECTORS

42

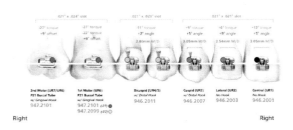

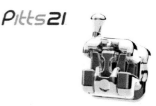

43   44

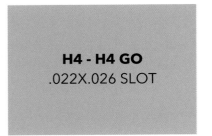

H4 - H4 GO
.022X.026 SLOT

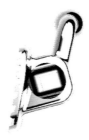

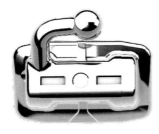

45

3. Archwire progression

In this case, we use an archwire progression made of 3 different alloys in the maxilla. *(Figs. 46 to 49)*

.014 **Niti Pitts Broad**
.018 x .018 **Niti Ultra Soft Pitts Broad**
.020 x .20 **Niti Pitts Broad**
.020 x .020 **B Titanio**
.019 x .019 **Acero**

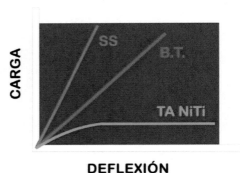

46

.014 **Niti Pitts Broad**
.018 x .018 **Niti Ultra Soft Pitts Broad**
.020 x .20 **Niti Pitts Broad**
.020 x .20 **Niti Ultrasoft Pitts Broad** (optional after Repo Appt)

47

Pitts21

48

ARCHWIRES
.020x.020 **BT Pitts Broad**
optional .019x.019 **SS Pitts Broad**
optional .020x.020 for extra with

49

For closing the large space, we selected the .019 x .019 steel archwire as its rigidity and low friction would allow an orderly movement in a 11mm gap.

4. Disarticulations
5. Elastics

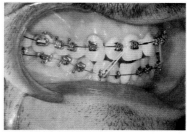 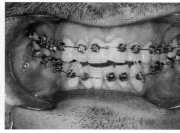 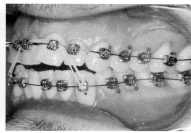

50   51   52

Images 50 to 52 show the newly installed appliance with a .014 NiTi Pitts Broad archwire, but with some particularities.

A) Although tooth # 16 was going to be extracted, a tube was bonded to the molar, using it as part of the transversal development of the upper arch.

B) Due to the periodontal condition of the lower incisor-canine sector, we performed interproximal reductions (IPR) of 2 mm in said sector.

Initially, no attachment was adhered to tooth # 41 and a «baby eyelet» was bonded to tooth # 42, aiming for reducing the .014 NiTi load/deflection even more.

C) Posterior disarticulations and isometric muscle exercise (squeezing) of the mandibular elevator muscles began.

D) The use of ILSE started with 5/16" 2.5 oz rainbow elastics in anterior teeth.

E) «Lingual reminders» bonding was rescheduled for the next session.

Weeks later, the .018 x .018 NiTi Ultra Soft Pitts Broad was installed, which was cut at the level of tooth # 16, keeping a small posterior sectional involving the upper right third and second molars.
In the mandibular arch, we continued with .014 NiTi Pitts Broad archwire, but now with lower Pitts21 brackets of standard prescription (-6°) in all teeth. *(Figs. 53 to 54)*

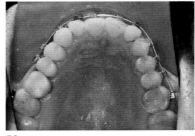 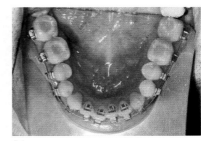

53   54

The next step was to install .020 x .020 NiTi Pitts Broad on the upper arch, where a «by pass» can be seen in tooth # 16.

The lower archwire changed to .018 x .018 NiTi Ultra Soft Pitts Broad.

The anterior rainbow elastic and neuromuscular exercise continued. *(Figs. 55 to 59)*

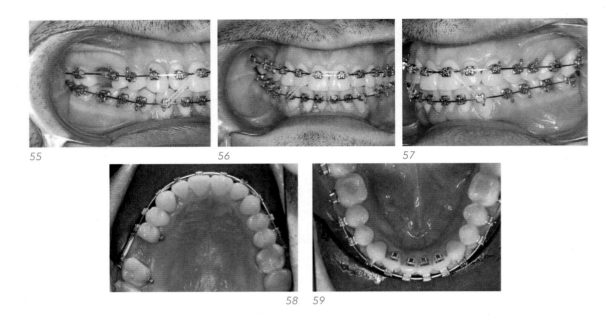

55   56   57

58   59

Before using an individualized .20 x .020 B Titanium, we switched to an archwire with greater rigidity but was somewhat smaller, such as the .019 x .019 steel archwire in which we «crimped» a post between premolars; from said attachment to the hook on tooth #18, we used a 12 mm NiTi closed coil spring with baby eyelets and 200 grams of force; this buccal closure force was regulated with an elastic chain placed between palatal buttons that were bonded to teeth # 18-17-15 and 14.
On the other hand, note that we insert an elastic chain between teeth # 15 and 25 above the .019 x .019 steel archwire in order to increase friction in all teeth except in # 18 and 17. *(Figs. 60 a 67)*

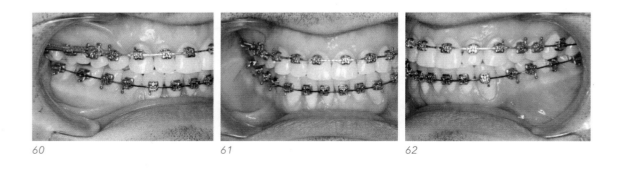

60   61   62